INFORMED CONSENT

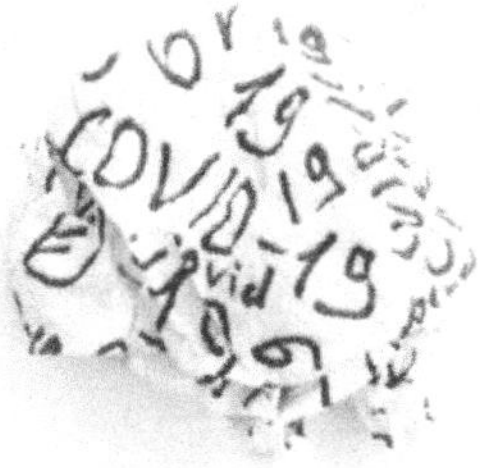

Exposing the Eugenics Cult:

& Their Latest Experiment on Mankind: COVID-19

Written by: Umm Nadia, Taliah S. Muhammad
Islamic Medicine Practitioner

Divine Ayat Publications, LLC
P.O. Box 29004
Henrico, Virginia 23242.

ISBN 978-1-7370880-0-4
ISBN 978-1-7370880-1-1 (eBook)

Table of Contents

Contents

Introduction

ALWAYS SPEAK THE TRUTH

بسمله الرحمن الرحيم

In the name of Allah, The Most Gracious,
The Most Merciful

All praise is to Allah, we praise Him and we seek His help and His forgiveness. We seek refuge with Allah from the evil of our own souls and from our bad deeds, whomsoever Allah guides will never be led astray; and whomsoever is led astray, no one can guide. I bear witness that none has the right to be worshiped but Allah, alone with no partner or associate, and that Muhammad (ﷺ) is His slave and His Messenger. ‘O you who believe! Fear Allah as He should be feared, and die not except in the state of Islam as Muslims with complete submission to Allah.’ And: ‘O mankind! Be dutiful to your Lord, Who created you from a single person, and from him He created his wife, and from them both He created many men and women, and fear Allah through Whom you demand your mutual (rights), and (do not cut the relations of) the wombs (kinship). Surely, Allah is Ever an All-Watcher over you.’ And: ‘O you who believe! Keep your duty to Allah and fear Him, **and speak (always) the truth**. He will direct you to do righteous good deeds and will forgive you your sins.’

(Sunan Ibn Majah, 1892)

Informed Consent

"Informed consent involves providing a potential subject with adequate information to allow for an informed decision about participation in the clinical investigation, facilitating the potential subject's comprehension of the information, providing adequate opportunity for the potential subject to ask questions and to consider whether to participate, obtaining the potential subject's voluntary agreement to participate, and continuing to provide information as the clinical investigation progresses or as the subject or situation requires. To be effective, the process must provide sufficient opportunity for the subject to consider whether to participate."

-U.S. Food & Drug Administration, (21 CFR 50.20.)

This work is the culmination of a yearlong study into the pathophysiology of COVID-19, though I dare to call it that as I feel my work has truly just begun. My inquiry into this dis-ease started haphazardly, or at least as my narrow mindedness would then perceive it, though my heart felt divinely inspired from the onset. My then three-year-old son was experiencing an ear infection which was characterized by fluid behind his eardrum. As an Herbalist, my goal was to find a remedy suitable for his condition. Despite my best efforts, the ear infection persisted.

At some point, I began to research "chronic ear infections" and this led to my now comfortable acquaintance with a bacterium called Nontypeable Haemophilus Influenza or NTHi. Coupled with Divine Signs from Allah, fear was also a catalyst for my headlong engrossment in the world of pathogenic bacteria. As I would learn, NTHi is a frequent cause of otitis media or recurring ear infections in children and has life-threatening consequences should it become invasive.

NTHi is a quite common gram-negative coccobacillus that colonizes the nasopharyngeal region in up to 80% of all humans. It is present in the nose and throat of 50% of all children and is usually harmless until it moves into the middle ear or the lungs where it can become fatal. After discovering that young boys like my son are more prone to chronic ear infections, I was thrust upon a path to learn all I could about NTHi.

My research into NTHi started sometime in late March or early April of 2020. Either way, I do remember it being a short time after the World Health Organization (WHO) declared COVID-19 a pandemic on March 11, 2020. Discovering that an invasive NTHi infection could spread to the lungs in conjunction with WHO declaring COVID-19 a respiratory virus was frightening, as the prognosis of a person having both dis-eases simultaneously did not seem promising.

Through my research, I found that patients colonized with

NTHi may be at risk for severe dis-ease as specific viruses, like COVID-19, on top of a bacterial infection may significantly enhance the risk for excessive inflammation which is also known as a "cytokine storm". Cytokine storm leads to the rapid formation of millions of foreign cells which attack the body through epithelial and endothelial tissues. This can cause a wide range of clinical presentations including systemic blood clotting, stroke, acquired hemolytic anemia, Kawasaki dis-ease, heart attack, and rapid cancer- all of which are symptoms found in patients with severe COVID-19 infections. It was at this discovery, that what started out as an Herbalist attempting to find a natural remedy for her sons' ear infection turned into full-blown COVID-19 research.

In an effort to inform others, I quickly released a two-hour long YouTube video on April 25, 2020 which documented some of my preliminary findings. Not everyone whom I shared the video with took part in my enthusiasm for this research. Thus, the too long video filled with my scientific ramblings received less than 20 views if my recollection serves me well. Eventually, I decided to shorten the video to 22 minutes precisely and the viewership increased to around 300 before its eventual takedown many months later. Still, it seemed no one paid much attention to my warnings that chronic ear infections may be a marker of COVID-19 contagiousness in children.

There were many moments during my nightlong research escapades, which were filled with coffee drinking, highlighting, and many "ahh haa" moments, that I questioned myself in the solace and quiet of the darkness. I knew I was being led by Allah, The Most High, to complete this task but why wasn't anyone listening? What exactly was I supposed to be doing all with this information? What was I missing?

Looking back however, I am glad my videos did not get much attention. Firstly, much of the science connecting NTHi and COVID-19 remained elusive to me. Though, I knew intuitively the relationship was present, there was still so much information that I needed in order to paint the parallel in adequate detail. As I have come to realize, scientific research unfolds just as patiently, methodically, and beautifully as my beloved chamomile flower does at sunrise.

Secondly, as my research progressed, so did a growing notion that the connection between NTHi and the emergence of COVID-19 could in no way be coincidental. In other words, the COVID-19 pandemic had to have been planned by man. Though, once again, there was much Allah, The Most High, had yet to show me so I could make this connection with proof. Had I come out with these assumptions without scientific proof, my claims would surely seem to others to be the mere speculation of a theorist with conspiracies.

As I continued my research, it occurred to me that the videos needed to be taken down and my thoughts should be collected in a concise form. Thus, emerged my research paper entitled; "COVID-19: The Plague That Strikes Behind the Ear". Initially, I made attempts to publish my research in major journals, but all these efforts were futile. In truth, I did not expect much from this process as the paper is written based upon an Islamic point of view, which to be clear, is the only *true* point of view. As Muslims, we know that there are many who reject Islam and though my science may resonate with some of these Darwinian academics, the mention of the name of Allah, The Most High, too often does not. May Allah, The Exalted, keep us safe from this tragedy, Ameen.

As a result, I decided to self-publish my research via my website, www.DivineAyat.com , ResearchGate, and Academia on January 1st, 2021. Though it was almost a year later, and still my research did not seem to be garnishing much attention, the motivation to press forward occurred when I came across other research linking chronic ear infections to COVID-19.

The first of that research was published by a researcher named Mihaela Chialda who worked at Sibiu County Emergency Clinical Hospital in Romania. The title the paper read; "ACUTE MASTOIDITIS- BEGINNING OF COVID-19 INFECTION – CASE REPORT". For reference, mastoiditis is considered a dis-ease of the middle ear and is the result of infection. I was stunned as I read parts of the abstract which detailed Chialdas' experience with a 59-year-old female patient. She had come into the emergency room complaining of "intense constrictive headaches" with no other symptoms. The patient was then given a series of test to include a CT scan which revealed right mastoiditis. She was then admitted to the emergency department and twenty-four hours later she tested positive for COVID-19. Chilada noted; "*The presence of the virus in the middle ear is almost constant even if the patient is asymptomatic.*" (1)

This research most certainly would have been cited in my paper had it not been published in the ACTA Medica Transilvanica Journal on January 28, 2021, a month after I formally published my research. At this point, that did not matter. What mattered was my research now had validation, Alhamdullilah. Whilst I was on one side of the world connecting the 'theoretical dots' between ear infections and COVID-19, Allah, The Most High, had a researcher in another part of the world verifying this connection in a 59-year-old patient.

I would soon learn that Chialda and I were not the only ones in the world calling the medical community to pay attention to the middle ear as it relates to COVID-19 infectivity. Several other case studies from researchers from hospitals in Turkey, Iran, and the United States (including Johns Hopkins University and The University of Virginia) had all published research on this link, with actual case studies (2-5) though none of the research pointed specifically to NTHi.

To date, it remains unclear exactly how COVID-19 emerged despite the half-hearted efforts by WHO to conduct a study in Wuhan, China almost one year after the beginning of the pandemic. It was perplexing to see how unprepared world governments were despite receiving "warnings" of a looming pandemic for years. Listening to President Trump chatter on about using ultraviolet rays and bleach solutions internally as possible treatments for COVID-19 was even more confusing. At the same time, I along with the rest disoriented public, watched the race to develop vaccines, and not just any vaccines – mRNA vaccines. Despite being a technology that has never been approved for use on the general public before, the mRNA vaccines were rushed through clinical trials and given Emergency Use Authorizations. These things along with other strange occurrences (that I will discuss later) encouraged my investigation into the NTHi – COVID-19 connection by Allah's Permission.

Deeper research took me on amazing excursions through books, videos, and scientific journals I had never traversed before. During one such exploration I came upon a stockpile of information on the topic of Eugenics. Surveying its contents was fascinating.

Eugenics can be defined as a biological and social science movement which promotes and facilitates the use of practices designed at improving the genetic composition of a society. Historically, Eugenics has been practiced for millennia by many elite societies including ancient Greece, Sparta, and the Roman empire, among others. The basic themes of this movement include the notions that there is an elite group who should bear the responsibility of government leadership and the protection of society. Additionally, this group believes it has an obligation to ensure the survival of the "fittest" members of society. To Eugenicists, these persons include those who are wealthy, intelligent, law abiding, physically strong, healthy, and those who possess other desirable characteristics which would contribute to a progressive and thriving society. Furthermore, this elite group believes that it must protect the demise of society (and the world for that matter), by identifying, controlling, and ultimately *eliminating* groups with undesirable characteristics which would necessarily include those who are poor, less intelligent, unhealthy, cowardly, criminal and so on.

Though, some form of Eugenics has been practiced for thousands of years, the actual term "Eugenics" was coined in 1883 by a man named Sir Francis Galton, who was an English proponent of eugenics and scientific racism. Speaking before the Sociological Society in 1904, Galton defined Eugenics as both a *science* and a *religion*. He encouraged his fellow eugenicists, who were also members of the scientific community, to *study and disseminate important knowledge on heredity* - which is how physical or mental characteristics are passed on genetically from one generation to another. He believed that each race should be represented by its "best specimens" and that understanding genetics might give future eugenicists a *scientific advantage* in creating a strong and powerful society.

In 1909, five years after Galton's call to study heredity, a Danish scientist named Wilhelm Johannsen coined the term "gene" to describe a basic unit of heredity which includes DNA and RNA (6). Eugenicist knew then that in order to manipulate DNA, they would have to learn more about its structure. One year later in 1910, Cold Spring Harbor Laboratory, a research facility in New York, began to dive into the study of eugenics by establishing the Eugenics Record Office (ERO) making New York the hub of the American Eugenics Movement (7). The ERO would go on to produce research on genetic differences between races, particularly making comparisons of the genetic differences between those deemed intelligent and those determined to be criminal (8).

After years of long research, scientists James Watson and Francis Crick would uncover the structure of DNA in 1953 (9). With this discovery arose many new scientific inquiries into the *sequence* of DNA. Essentially, now that the structure of DNA was discovered, it became essential for Eugenicists to know the specific "codes" of DNA so that editing the code could be made precisely and without error. *It must be noted, that much of this research was made under the guise of understanding and curing heritable dis-ease.*

To discover the sequence of DNA, The Cold Spring Harbor Laboratory would launch the Human Genome Project in 1990. This project ran for 13 years, (until 2003) and was part of the International Human Genome Sequencing Consortium, a collection of labs and organizations located in America, France, Germany, Japan, China, and the United Kingdom. It was funded by the National Human Genome Research Institute, The National Institutes of Health (NIH), The U.S. Department of Energy (DOE), and the Wellcome Trust in London, UK (10).

In 1998, the U.S. Human Genome Project, under the direction of Francis Collins (who is now the Director of the National Institutes of Health), would set specific goals. One of those goals included the development of a genetics-based technology that would change the way medicines would be administered in the future. According to their plan, this research might include "creating mutations that cause a loss or alteration of function in order to study gene function which could be performed in both cell lines and whole organisms, including humans" (11).

The consortium met their first goal of discovering sequence of DNA which would lead to yet another greedy inquiry; now *that DNA is sequenced, how can it be edited?* Not all scientist at the time were convinced that DNA was the key to editing the human genome. A small group of scientists at Harvard University thought that RNA might be the key to changing the genetic code.

Upon learning all this, I began to ponder much over the connection between gene editing via RNA interference, a subject I had a basic familiarity with, and the new mRNA vaccines for COVID-19. I decided that taking hard look into the research projects at the Cold Spring Harbor Laboratory, particularly those performed under the Human Genome Project, might be the key in making the connection between the two. It was through this analysis that I became familiar with the research of Jennifer Doudna, a mentee of James Watson. Doudna spent much of her career studying the structure of RNA. She and her colleagues would go on to discover its structure and publish their findings in a research paper in *Science* in September of 1996 (12). What I found particularly interesting is that Doudna did not just study RNA, much of her research included studying how the RNA in coronaviruses, allow them to highjack the protein making systems of cells (13). Through her research she found that coronaviruses could hack into human cells and change the way proteins behave and in 2012, she would co-create CRISPR-Cas9, a gene editing technology that can be used to change the human genome.

Though all this information was interesting and seemed quite relevant, one question still loomed over me; *how does all this relate to NTHi*? That question would be answered when I learned about *bacteriophages.* Some viruses called bacteriophages or "phage" for short, specifically target bacteria like NTHi. Uncoincidentally, bacteriophages were a major topic of study at the Cold Spring Harbor Laboratory, in fact, they ran a course there on bacteriophages for over 25 years (14). What really put things in perspective is when I learned that NTHi is the gateway to many important gene clusters and if they were to become altered, it would cause evolutionary changes in the human genome (15).

The NTHi – COVID-19 connection now became clearer: COVID-19 is the moment that modern Eugenicists have been striving for since the turn of the 19th century: <u>genetic advantage of the "elite" over all others.</u> Due the presence of NTHI in over half of the world's population, it makes this opportunistic bacterium a perfect target for a gene editing experiment *in vivo*.

It is my firm belief that COVID-19 is a highly orchestrated and deliberate attempt by the Cult of Eugenics to practice their Darwinian beliefs of survival of the fittest, selective racism, and intervening into natural selection on mankind. It is my vehement desire to expose their evil plots in shaa Allah.

My purpose for writing this book is simple, I do not believe that the public has been informed about this public health crisis we call COVID-19 in terms of its origin and further, its purpose. Consequently, do not I believe that the public has enough information to make a valid informed decision about taking the mRNA COVID-19 vaccines. My goal is to provide you with scientifically based information so that you can confidently form your opinions about COVID-19 and ultimately the necessity for the COVID-19 vaccines with sound knowledge.

Since the accurate conveyance of this type of information can be a bit technical and overly scientific at times, I have made my best attempts in presenting the material in a straightforward way so even if one is not given to scientific research, they can still enjoy the nuances of the subjects I enjoy including Pathophysiology, Microbiology, Genetics, and foremost Islamic Medicine.

Much of the research to be explained later in this work builds upon my research paper; "COVID-19: The Plague that Strikes Behind the Ear." To fully understand the concepts that will be presented later, I have decided it necessary to publish the full research in the first chapter of this work. I think you will find it beneficial to read the research paper first, but I see equal benefit in starting to read at the second chapter and saving chapter one for last.

If there is anything good in this work, then know that all good comes from Allah, The Most High. If there are any errors, then surely it is from myself. May Allah, The Most High, guide you, forgive you, and grant you provision. Ameen.

Umm Nadia, Taliah S. Muhammad

Ramadan 29, 1442 AH

Chapter One

COVID-19: THE PLAGUE THAT STRIKES BEHIND THE EAR

Review

COVID-19: The Plague that Strikes Behind the Ear

Taliah Safah Muhammad[1,2,*]

[1]Divine Ayat, LLC., Henrico, P.O. Box 29004, Henrico, Virginia 23242.
[2]Halal Natural Products Academy, LLC., Henrico, Virginia.

ABSTRACT

Nontypeable Haemophilus Influenzae (NTHI) is a major cause of invasive dis-ease worldwide. Viral infections in patients colonized with NTHI may be at risk for serious complications as specific viruses, like SAR-CoV-2, on top of a bacterial infection significantly enhances the risk for excessive inflammation and upregulation of ICAM-1. ICAM-1 is elevated in COVID-19 patients with mild dis-ease and dramatically elevated in severe cases. C-C chemokine receptor CCR5 is also upregulated in COVID-19 patients. Incidentally, ICAM-1 and CCR5 upregulation are both implicated in the pathogenesis and progression of HIV. Like the HIV, SARS-CoV-2 gains cellular entry through CD4 T-cells. A NTHI / SARS-CoV-2 co-infection causes LFA-1 binding to ICAM-1. LFA-1 activation on target CD4 T-cells enhances SARS-CoV-2 infectivity and transmission by promoting virus binding and cell to cell spread via the CCR5 coreceptor. These mechanisms allow SARS-CoV-2 cellular access to multiple cellular systems inducing a cytokine storm in some patients. LFA-1also increases the cell susceptibility to bacterial toxin LtxA that preferentially targets active LFA-1. Leukotoxin (LtxA; Leukothera), is a protein toxin secreted by the oral bacterium Aggregatibacter actinomy cetemcomitans, which specifically kills white blood cells. Interestingly, Aggregatibacter actinomycetemcomitans and NTHI are two species under genus Pasteurellaceae. Throughout history, plagues have been associated with divine punishments from God caused by bacterias. Prophet Muhammadﷺ told us over 1400 years ago that when fornication becomes widespread new dis-eases like COVID-19 would increase. A holistic approach including Spiritual, Physical, Emotional, and Mental interventions must be employed to treat COVID-19 as well as to prevent the next pandemic.

Keywords: NTHI , Plague, COVID-19, CCR5, ICAM-1, HIV/AIDS

1. Introduction

For Muslims, Islam is a complete way of life that promotes homeostasis in the Spiritual, Physical, Mental, and Emotional domains of wellness. COVID-19 has thrust this generation into a very precarious time where understanding and exploring Islamic pathways to wellness is obviously more relevant now than ever. For example, key principles to promote wellness during COVID-19 include; social distancing which entails refraining from handshaking, an emphasis on physical cleanliness through frequent handwashing, and covering the face and hands, which are all fundamental acts performed daily by billions of Muslims all over the world as religious obligations.

The Islamic approach to medicine is "holistic" as it puts forth that Spiritual, Physical (to include the use of whole plant medicine), Mental, and Emotional causes of dis-ease must be identified and properly treated in order to open the pathway for a complete cure. Treating symptoms is a common approach that may slow one dis-ease progression while acting as a catalyst for another thus, it does not lead to a complete cure. This can be exemplified in the case of the overprescription of antibiotics for dis-eases like STDs. The overprescription of antibiotics for dis-eases like STDs led to antibiotic resistant bacteria such as NTHI and Candida albicans. This can also be evidenced in the decrease in the incidence of invasive Hib dis-eases due to widespread use of the Hib vaccine. Consequently, NTHi strains have taken the lead in becoming the most common cause of invasive dis-ease in all age groups with routine Hib vaccination (1).

Prophet Muhammadسلى الله عليه و سلم, (may the peace and blessings of Allah be upon him) told us the reasons why we would experience new dis-eases like COVID-19;

"...If fornification should become widespread, you should realize that this has never happened without new dis-eases befalling the people which their forebears never suffered." (2).

We are indeed living in a time where fornication has become widespread and deemed morally acceptable by a majority. Results from a 2002 U.S. survey revealed that by age 20, 75% of all respondents had premarital sex. It further revealed that by age 44, 95% of respondents (94% of women, 96% of men, and 97% of those who had ever had sex) had had premarital sex. The conclusions of this survey by the National Survey of Family Growth indicated that almost all Americans have sex before marrying (3).

According to a 2019 Pew Research Study, 62% of respondents in the U.S. said casual sex between consenting adults who aren't in a committed relationship is acceptable at least sometimes (4).

Another survey conducted by The Pew Research Center in 2014 compared global views of premarital sex found that respondents in predominantly Muslim countries like Indonesia, Jordan, Turkey and Egypt overwhelmingly agreed that premarital sex is morally wrong. Western countries such as Europe mainly found premarital sex morally acceptable (4).

What is a plague?

According to the Merriam Webster Dictionary, the word plague has several meanings. For one, it can mean a disastrous evil or affliction. It can also mean a virulent contagious febrile dis-ease that is caused by a bacterium (Yersinia pestis) and that occurs in bubonic, pneumonic, and septicemic forms.

Islam is a complete way of life. The Qur'an (The Speech of Allah) and Sunnah (legal ways of Prophet Muhammad سلى الله عليه و سلم) provide mankind with knowledge needed to achieve wellness and a cure Spiritually, Physically, Mentally, and Emotionally. When mankind accepts this knowledge given by Allah and then acts upon it, they are given the opportunity to achieve holistic wellness. When societies act in opposition to the Qur'an and Sunnah it opens the pathways to sickness and ultimately death which is brought on by widespread calamities, fitna and trials.

<u>Allah سُبۡحَانَهُۥ وَتَعَالَىٰ says in The Qur'an;</u>

يَٰٓأَيُّهَا ٱلَّذِينَ ءَامَنُواْ ٱسۡتَجِيبُواْ لِلَّهِ وَلِلرَّسُولِ إِذَا دَعَاكُمۡ لِمَا يُحۡيِيكُمۡۖ وَٱعۡلَمُوٓاْ أَنَّ ٱللَّهَ يَحُولُ بَيۡنَ ٱلۡمَرۡءِ وَقَلۡبِهِۦ وَأَنَّهُۥٓ إِلَيۡهِ تُحۡشَرُونَ

وَٱتَّقُواْ فِتۡنَةٗ لَّا تُصِيبَنَّ ٱلَّذِينَ ظَلَمُواْ مِنكُمۡ خَآصَّةٗۖ وَٱعۡلَمُوٓاْ أَنَّ ٱللَّهَ شَدِيدُ ٱلۡعِقَابِ

"Oh you who believe! Answer Allah (by obeying Him) and (His) Messenger سلى الله عليه و سلم when He calls you to that which will give you life, and know that Allah comes in between and person and his heart (i.e. He prevents an evil person from deciding anything). And verily, to Him you shall

(all) be gathered.

And fear the *Fitnah* (affliction and trial) which affects not in particular (only) those of you who do wrong (but it may afflict all the good and the bad people), and know that Allah is Severe in punishment." **Surah Al-Anfal, 8:24-25** (*The Noble Qur'an*) (5).

Ibn Qiyyum رحمه الله a renowned scholar in Islam stated in his book; "Medicine of The Prophet":

"Although the plague describes every infection that sends septic blood to the heart, becoming fatal sometimes, it particularly describes the infection that attacks the soft tissues of the body. Since the infected blood is septic, the various organs reject the blood, except those that have become weak. The worst types of plague are those that strike behind the ears and under the arms, because they are closer to the essential organs of the body." (6).

According to the CDC, there are three types of plague: bubonic, septicemic, and pneumonic. In pneumonic plague patients develop fever, headache, weakness, and a rapidly developing pneumonia with shortness of breath, chest pain, cough, and sometimes bloody or watery mucus. Pneumonic plague may develop from inhaling infectious droplets or may develop from untreated bubonic or septicemic plague after the bacteria spread to the lungs. The pneumonia may cause respiratory failure and shock. Pneumonic plague is the most serious form of the dis-ease and is the only form of plague that can be spread from person to person (by infectious droplets) (7).

Symptoms presented by COVID-19 patients strongly resemble symptoms of pneumonic plague to include shortness of breath, fever, headache, tiredness, cough, and Pneumonia (8).

2. Nontypeable Haemophilus Influenzae (NTHI): The Bacteria Behind the New Plague

According to research on emerging pathogens published by the National Institutes of Health in 2015, Nontypeable Haemophilus Influenzae (NTHI) is a major cause of invasive dis-ease worldwide (9). It is believed that this emergence may be partly due to increased NTHi colonization in children which might contribute to increased transmission to persons susceptible to developing invasive NTHi dis-ease. Over the last 25 years in the U.S., the elderly have accounted for 89% of all invasive NTHI infections. Much like SARS-CoV-2, pre-existing dis-eases such as COPD, cancer, chronic renal failure, and diabetes place people at greater risk for contracting invasive NTHI (10, 11). However, it has been found that NTHI infections are not just found in persons with immunocompromising conditions or co-existing conditions but in almost half the cases in persons who were otherwise in good health (11).

Viral infections in patients colonized with NTHI may be at risk for future exacerbations as specific viruses, like SAR-CoV-2, on top of a bacterial infection may significantly enhance the risk for excessive inflammation. In a 2015 study, it was found that Nontypeable Haemophilus influenzae (NTHI) can enhance expression of the cellular receptor intercellular adhesion molecule 1 (ICAM-1) on airway epithelial cells, which in turn increases the binding of major group human rhinoviruses (HRVs) for attachment (12).

Major group human rhinoviruses or HRVs are members of the Picornaviridae family. Like Coronaviruses or CoVs, they are a large family of single stranded RNA viruses. These viruses can cross species barriers and can cause, in humans, illness ranging from the common cold to more severe diseases such as MERS and SARS (13).

Many COVID-19 patients experience symptoms that are similar to symptoms presented by those who have COPD including frequent coughing, excess phlegm, shortness of breath, and trouble breathing (8). Recent studies have focused on the role of viral and bacterial coinfection in patients with COPD. This coinfection is associated with incidences of intensified respiratory dis-ease and more inflammation (14). The most common co-infection is with rhinovirus (RV) and NTHI in COPD (15-16). NTHI also has significant and scientifically noted high morbidity risks for patients who smoke, or have Bronchiectasis, Cystic Fibrosis, Pneumonia, and Intestinal Lung Dis-ease (17). These factors and dis-eases are also associated with increased risk of severe complications from COVID-19 (10).

NTHI is a very common gram-negative coccobacillus that colonizes the nasopharyngeal region in up to 80% of humans (18). It is present in the nose and throat of 50% of all children and is usually harmless until it moves to the middle ear or the lungs where it can cause the most damage. NTHI is a frequent cause of otitis media (chronic middle ear infections) (19) in children and acute bronchitis and pneumonia in patients with chronic obstructive pulmonary dis-ease (20). Non-typeable Haemophilus influenzae (NTHI) has been associated with early pregnancy loss and in a 2020 report it was deemed an emerging neonatal and maternal pathogen (21).

This bacterium needs an iron rich environment to survive. Once NTHI has moved into the lungs and middle ear, heme iron is sequestered as part of the body's immune response. Instead of dying, the bacterium is kept alive by using clever hacks of the host's immune response (22).

Scientists Kevin M. Mason, PhD and Sheryl S. Justice, PhD, principal investigators in the Center for Microbial Pathogenesis figured out how NTHI was able to maintain a relatively low profile amongst clinicians with respiratory/pulmonary backgrounds and not be considered an important pathogenic bacterium. Their research shows that NTHI uses the body's own immune system to its advantage. Once the immune system is alerted of a bacterial invasion in the lungs, middle ear, and other parts of the body, the immune system cuts off access to nutrients the bacteria need to survive- including heme iron. This process is known as nutritional immunity. This immune response triggers a series of additional immune defenses to include inflammation, which involves the release of chemicals that are designed to find and sequester NTHI and bring in white blood cells to the site of infection to destroy the invading bacterium (22).

The scientist developed a lab experiment designed to imitate the immune response to NTHI infection in the middle ear and to further observe how NTHI responds to the body's immune responses. The research results showed that in the body's immune response a serum designed to carry dis-ease fighting chemicals and white blood cells to the site of the infection includes heme-iron. They further observed that when NTHI was re-exposed to heme-iron the bacteria underwent structural changes that allowed it to divide much more slowly and become elongated and spaghetti-like in appearance. As a result, the NTHI was ignored by the dis-ease fighting white blood cells as they usually target rapidly dividing shorter cells. Thus, NTHI was left alone to replicate and thrive. "This clearly shows that NTHI is changing to become more fit in the host," says Dr. Justice, who also is an assistant professor of pediatrics and urology at the Ohio State University College of Medicine (23).

Much like NTHI, SARS-Co-V-2 also has the ability to block the host innate immune response through its links to the function of structural and non-structural proteins (24) which makes co-infection with invasive NTHI and SARS-Co-V-2 a severe threat to host morbidity. In three separate studies it was found that COVID-19 patients were co-infected with Haemophilus Influenzae (96-98).

3. Upregulated ICAM-1 in COVID-19 Patients Could be Due to NTHI + SARS-CoV-2 Co-Infections

To date it is believed that SARS-CoV-2 via its surface

spike glycoprotein interacts with Angiotensin-converting enzyme 2 (ACE2) and invades host cells. ACE2 is expressed in human vascular endothelium, respiratory epithelium, and other cell types (25). Endothelial cells play an important role in virtually every system in the body. These cells form the inner lining of the cardiovascular and lymphatic systems. They make up the inner layer of blood and lymphatic vessels and organs including the brain, lungs, skin and heart. Epithelial cells provide biochemical barriers by synthesizing and secreting substances meant to trap or destroy bacteria like NTHI (26). However, NTHI is able to allow its binding to epithelial cells. There is also evidence that NTHI may thrive in the respiratory tract by surviving inside of epithelial cells (27).

Though ACE2 is thought to be the main point of cellular entry for SARS-CoV-2, it is well known that viruses often use a variety of mechanisms for attachment. The most common cell adhesion molecules are CAMs which are routinely exploited by viruses to gain cellular entry (28). A retrospective study of COVID-19 patients in China found that serum levels of fractalkine, vascular cell adhesion molecule-1 (VCAM-1), intercellular adhesion molecule 1 (ICAM-1), and vascular adhesion protein-1 (VAP-1) were elevated in patients with mild dis-ease, dramatically elevated in severe cases, and decreased in the convalescence phase (29).

Much like Human herpesvirus 8 (HHV-8), HIV, and AIDS, NTHI can inhibit epithelial host defense proteins (30-33). Once compromised, airway epithelial cells respond to the invasion of NTHI by secreting inflammatory acute-phase reactants such as IL-6, IL-8, and TNF-ą (31,32). NTHI then increases the expression of ICAM-1 by airway epithelial cells which increases the susceptibility of viruses binding to the cells (34).

ICAM-1 or Intercellular Adhesion Molecule 1, also known as CD54 (Cluster of Differentiation) is a protein that in humans is encrypted by the ICAM-1 gene. The ICAM-1 gene is coded by a cell surface glycoprotein which is expressed on endothelial cells and cells of the immune system (35). An NTHI and SARS-CoV-2 co-infection that originates from the middle ear might allow these pathogens cellular access to the respiratory system as scientists have discovered that there is a similar allergic inflammation in the middle ear and the upper airway suggesting the middle ear may be a part of the united airways concept (36). The major leading cause of death in patients with COVID-19 is respiratory failure from acute respiratory distress syndrome (ARDS) (37).

4. Comparing the Pathophysiology of COVID-19 to that of HIV/AIDS for better understanding of the dis-ease and to develop treatments

Many receptors for cytokines/chemokines have recently been identified by a group of scientists as upregulated in COVID-19 patients including; C-C chemokine receptor (CCR) 1 (CCR1), CCR2, and CCR5. These same scientists claim; "our work highlights opportunities for clinical trials with existing or under development CCR5 drugs to treat high risk or severe COVID-19 cases" (38). ICAM-1 and CCR5 upregulation are both implicated in the pathogenesis and progression of HIV (39, 40).

It has been previously established that HIV's replication is facilitated by ICAM-1 which is believed to increase infection of CD4 T-cells (41). Plasma biomarkers of endothelial injury such as higher levels of cICAM-1, lower levels of cICAM2, an increase in cB2 microglobulin levels, and the decrease in CD4 T-cell counts are well established predictive biomarkers in HIV1-infected patients used to determine dis-ease progression and prognosis for AIDS progression (39). These same markers may be useful in determining dis-ease progression and prognosis in asymptomatic COVID-19 patients and further identifying potential therapeutic candidates.

Due to the similarities between COVID-19 and HIV dis-ease infection and progression, a closer look at the mechanisms of HIV infection is warranted. HIV gains entry into the cells via gp120 and CD4. This allows for binding to the chemokine receptors CCR5 or CXCR4, which act as coreceptors for the virus for which CD4 antibodies have been identified as effective therapeutic targets (42). It is important to note that a 2008 research study found that HIV transfer between CD4 T-cells did not require LFA-1 binding to ICAM-1 and is governed by the interaction of HIV envelope glycoprotein with CD4. The researchers discovered that HIV transmission between infected and uninfected primary CD4 T-cells was stopped by inhibitors of gp120 binding to CD4 by not blocking LFA-1 binding to ICAM-1 or ICAM-3. Further, it was noted that LFA-1 and ICAM-3 monoclonal antibodies (MoAb) actually enhanced HIV transfer (43). Recent research noted that CCR5 receptor and chromosome 3 gene clusters contribute to susceptibility to COVID-19 and the development of severe complications. Additionally, delta-32 allele , a polymorphism in CCR5 that regulates its expression has been identified as a partial to full protection against HIV infection and acts as a foundational basis for gene deletion studies aimed at achieving a permanent cure to HIV (44-45). It should be noted that a positive correlation between COVID-19 mortality rate and the delta -32 allele in African population was found (46).

Further, there is a correlation between the progression of HIV and invasive NTHI infections. A study designed to evaluate increases in invasive NTHI infection from 2017-2018 among homosexual HIV infected men in Atlanta, Georgia found the incidence of invasive NTHI infection increased significantly from 2017-2018 compared with 2008-2016. Additionally, two unique but genetically connected strains were observed and associated with septic arthritis among homosexual black men who lived in geographic proximity (47).

On a spiritual level, it makes sense that there are such similarities between COVID-19 and HIV/AIDS as both have causes tied to fornication.

5. COVID-19 Pathophysiology may be much like HIV/AIDS with Distinct Characteristics

Like HIV, SARS-CoV-2 gains cellular entry via CD4 T-cells. However, different mechanisms lead to SARS-CoV-2 infection.

Asymptomatic people may be super spreaders of COVID-19 due to high levels of NTHI. SARS-CoV-2 rarely causes serious dis-ease super spreader populations yet, the virus causes severe dis-ease progression in others. This may be due to the condition of the innate immune system. Several groups have found that the binding of IgM to the bacterial surface might play a role in the innate defense against NTHI infections. Another study found that patients with hyper-IgM syndrome were less susceptible to NTHI colonization, a finding that emphasizes the role of IgM in the immune system defense against NTHI. The percentages of IgM-producing CD27+ memory B cells in the peripheral blood of children are low but increases to almost 20% in adults and declines again in the elderly. This might address the question of whether a diminished protective immunoglobulin level in the elderly contributes to susceptibility to invasive NTHI dis-ease (9).

The COVID-19 Model

1. A person with increased NTHI colonization becomes infected with SARS-CoV-2.
2. Due to a weakened immune system (lower IgM levels) the body pushes harder against the co-infection through mounting an excessive inflammatory response.
3. ICAM-1 becomes upregulated.
4. ICAM-1 acts as a ligand to LFA-1.
5. LFA-1 becomes activated on CD4 T-cells.

6. LFA-1 activation on target and infected CD4 T-cells enhance SARS-CoV-2 infectivity and transmission by promoting virus binding and cell to cell spread via the CCR5 coreceptor.

7. LFA-1also increases the cell susceptibility to bacterial toxin LtxA that preferentially targets active LFA-1 (48).

- Leukotoxin (LtxA; Leukothera), a protein toxin secreted by the oral bacterium Aggregatibacter actinomycetemcomitans, specifically kills white blood cells (WBCs). LtxA binds to the receptor known as lymphocyte function associated antigen-1 (LFA-1), a β2 integrin expressed only on the surface of WBCs (49).
- NTHI and Aggregatibacter actinomycetemcomitans are two species under genus Pasteurellaceae thus closely related (50).
- A. actinomycetemcomitans is associated with oral and non-oral dis-eases (51).

8. LtxA binds to the active form of LFA-1 and nominally affects cells that express resting-state LFA-1 (52-54). The mechanism of cellular killing by LtxA has been studied in HL-60 monocytes. It has been found that LtxA causes necrosis at high doses by forming pores in the host cell membrane, while at low doses LtxA induces apoptosis (55-56). This might explain why persons with increased NTHI and Aggregatibacter actinomycetemcomitans

colonization would be at a higher risk of severe complications from COVID-19.

6. Intestinal Dis-ease as a Marker for COVID-19 Dis-ease Progression

Prophet Muhammad, may peace and blessings be upon him, said, "The son of Adam cannot fill a vessel worse than his stomach, as it is enough for him to take a few bites to straighten his back. If he cannot do it, then he may fill it with a third of his food, a third of his drink, and a third of his breath." (57) It is well known that overeating (gluttony), particularly on unhealthy foods, can cause an array of stomach and intestinal dis-eases. Eating Disorders (ED) including Binge Eating (BE) has been associated with imbalances in the gut flora compromising gut health and immune defense maintenance. These imbalances are negatively correlated with anxiety and depression scores (58).

Cytokine induced changes in mucin expression and *O*-glycosylation are likely involved in the pathogenesis and progression of inflammatory bowel dis-eases (IBD) such as ulcerative colitis and Crohn's dis-ease. Disrupted gut barrier integrity is at the heart of all inflammatory bowel dis-eases (59-60).

A recent study performed by researchers Giron, Dweep and others revealed severe COVID-19 is fueled by disrupted gut barrier Integrity. These researchers found that hospitalized COVID-19 patients had higher plasma levels of zonulin, (the only known physiological conciliator of tight junction permeability in the digestive tract), and were more likely to die. This progression of dis-ease was due to the ability of microbes to enter into the bloodstream causing systemic inflammation. The researchers also pointed that systemic inflammation caused by a lung infection can lead to a disruption of the gut barrier integrity leading to microbial translocation. Upon examining plasma glycomes, their research uncovered that translocation of glycan-degrading enzymes alter extraintestinal circulating high-mannose glycoform (HM-ICAM-1) (61). Further, in the inflamed gut of Crohn's Dis-ease and Ulcerative Colitis patients, 1CAM-1 is enhanced. Research points to HM-ICAM-1, ICAM-1 as a key therapeutic target for controlling leukocyte trafficking and endothelial inflammation (62,63).

7. Candida albicans: a Therapeutic Target

Some bacteria in the normal intestinal microbiome are opportunistic. Opportunistic bacteria like Candida albicans can overgrow due to prolonged treatment with broad-spectrum antibiotics (64). Broad-spectrum antibiotics are often prescribed to target pathogens sensitive to antimicrobial agents. However, other organisms such as Candida albicans that are resistant to the therapeutic intervention invate the unoccupied space and multiply rapidly. This occurrence is called Candidiasis or superinfection (65). In 2019 the CDC listed drug resistant Candida species in its Antimicrobial Resistance Threats Report, stating that many are resistant to antifungals used to treat them (66).

When Candida albicans overgrowth and the normal lining of the intestinal tract is damaged, the body can absorb yeast cells, particles of yeast, and various toxins (67). Candida accounts for 70-90% of all invasive fungal infections in hospitalized patients and is a leading cause for sepsis in critically ill patients. Additionally, administration of broad-spectrum antibiotics, central vascular catheters, diabetes mellitus, parenteral nutrition, mechanical ventilation, renal insufficiency, hemodialysis, colonization, antifungal prophylaxis, surgery, pancreatitis, and treatment with corticosteroids and chemotherapy were the most frequently identified risk factors for sepsis in patients with Candidiasis (68). Researchers have increasingly become aware of COVID-19 fungal co-infections. The main fungal pathogens for fungal co-infections in severe COVID-19 patients are Aspergillus and Candida albicans (69).

On April 24, 2020 a 67 year old COVID-19 patient presented oral mucosal lesions resembling late state herpetic recurrent oral lesions associated with candidiasis. He was admitted to the ICU for supplemental oxygen therapy. The patient's symptoms worsened, and doctors suspected pneumonia. The patient was placed on antibiotic regimens. On the twenty fourth day of hospitalization, dentists discovered white patches on the patient's tongue. He was prescribed antifungal medications and the patches cleared up. The patient was released from ICU two weeks later and was discharged from the hospital after forty-four days. (70)

It should be noted that Acute Acquired Hemolytic Anemia has been associated with Herpes Simplex Infection (71).

Hemolytic anemia is a blood disorder that occurs when your red blood cells are destroyed faster than they can be replaced. Severe hemolytic anemia can cause fever, chills, back pain, shock, irregular heartbeat, and cardiomyopathy in which the heart grows larger than normal (72).

8. NTHI, SARS-CoV-2, Intestinal Dis-ease & Inflammation: Making Sense of MIS in Children

Inflammation can modify the glycosylation pattern of glycolipids and glycoproteins. It is well known that the glycosylation of acute-phase proteins is subjected to marked changes during acute and chronic inflammation (73). The inflammatory response caused by ICAM-1 Upregulation and COVID-19 can lead to increased levels of pro-inflammatory cytokines in response to pathogens lead to a constant NF-κB activation resulting in an increased synthesis of pro-inflammatory cytokines, which contributes the vicious inflammatory cycle seen in patients with Kawasaki dis-ease and other systemic inflammation presentations (74-75).

NTHi strains cause mucosal infections, including otitis media, conjunctivitis, sinusitis, bronchitis, and pneumonia. Less commonly, these strains cause invasive dis-ease in children but account for half of the invasive infections in adults which may explain why children are less likely to become severely ill from COVID-19 (76).

On August 7, 2020 a report on Multisystem Inflammatory Syndrome in Children (MIS-C) was released by the U.S. Department of Health and Human Services and the

CDC. Clinical symptoms of patients included in this report included fever, rash, conjunctivitis, peripheral edema, gastrointestinal symptoms, shock, and elevated markers of inflammation and cardiac damage.

This report found that of the 570 children with COVID-19 related MIS-C, 25% of them were obese. 90% of them experienced gastrointestinal symptoms including abdominal pain, vomiting, and diarrhea. About 71% of them experienced dermatologic and mucocutaneous presentations including rash (55.3%) and mucocutaneous lesions (35.3%). Furthermore, 60.4% of these children had Elevated D-dimer levels indicating significant formation and breakdown of blood clots in the body. Researchers further found that it is often difficult to distinguish MIS-C from other conditions like severe COVID-19 and Kawasaki dis-ease. Hispanic and Black children made up 73% of this study (75).

Discussions:

Male children who are more prone to chronic ear infections may be more likely to be the asymptomatic super spreaders of COVID-19. High COVID-19 morbidity rates among men may be explained by a lifetime overuse of antibiotics (for chronic ear infections and other dis-eases) which may have led to imbalance in gut flora specifically candida albicans infection, and a disrupted gut barrier. Generally, Men are underdiagnosed for candida albicans infection. Men become more susceptible to this infection by using testosterone containing products as research strongly suggests that testosterone plays an important role in decreasing resistance to systemic C. albicans infection (77).

Published national and state data shows that persons of color might be more likely to become infected with SARS-CoV-2, the virus that causes COVID-19, experience more severe COVID-19–associated illness, including that requiring hospitalization, and have higher risk for death from COVID-19 (78) and pre-existing anemia may be a contributing factor. Pre-existing anemias, can worsen the symptoms of NTHI/COVID-19 Infections during the nutritional immunity stage. During this stage iron is sequestered as a first line defense strategy. However, iron is reintroduced to NTHI which causes sharp rises and falls in iron levels which can have severe clinical implications for those who suffer with iron deficient blood. Furthermore, acquired haemolytic anemia may develop after treatment with drugs such as quinine, sulphonamides, para-amino-salicylic acid, or it may follow infections caused by bacteria or viruses (71). In the case of a patient with pre-existing anemias getting infected with NTHI/COVID-19 could be deadly especially when the aforementioned treatments are used. In a 2013 study, it was found that Blacks have moderate to severe anemia almost three times more than whites and hispanics (79).

Doctors have reported that after NIV respiratory therapy, there is a sudden, unexpected worsening of symptoms in some patients. This often leads to intubation and invasive mechanical ventilation (13). This may be due in part to the fact that Nontypeable Haemophilus bacteria is an anaerobe. These types of pathogens die quickly when exposed to oxygen. The rapid decline in patients' health after NIV may be explained by the Herxheimer Reaction or "die off effect" of the NTHi bacteria dying quickly.

Infections caused by NTHI are chronic and similar to other bacterial infections that are difficult to treat (23) with antibiotics. Antibiotics further strengthen bacterial resistant microbes which in turns further disrupts the gut barrier integrity. "In essence, antibiotics progress COVID-19 disease manifestations leaving moderate to severe patients open to re-infection. In severe patients, antibiotic therapies can lead to death as in the case of Penicillin. Penicillin is known to cause hemolytic anemia which can lead to hemorrhaging, blood clots, heart failure, and stroke" (80).

What Practitioners Can Do Now:

1. Consider Antiviral therapies using iminosugar derivatives. Since ADCC is thought to play a role in protecting against initial infection and controlling progression of infection in HIV, 2G12 dimmers may be a possible therapy (81). 2G12 is a neutralizing human monoclonal antibody that has 3 possible combining sites. It has been identified as a possible antiviral therapy for various viruses (82). Studies also suggest that "2G12 competitively inhibits interactions between gp120's V3 loop and the tyrosine sulfate-containing CCR5 amino terminus, thereby reducing assembly of complexes that catalyze entry (83).

2. Cleanse Patient Gut - consider using enema treatments with antisense oligonucleotides as a short-term remedy to reduce intestinal inflammation and downregulate ICAM-1 (84-86). A holistic approach using herbs and lifestyle modifications will be necessary to prevent symptom relapse after therapy.

3. Consider Replenishing Gut Flora via exaggerated probiotic therapy.

4. Consider available therapies using iminosugar derivatives for Candida Albicans overgrowth.

5. Enlist Resident Nutritionists with backgrounds in Vitamin Therapy, microbiology, biochemistry etc. to help formulate the appropriate (and available) therapies given the considerations outlined in this research.

6. Non-clinical and Clinical Trials of holistic Islamic Medicine Therapies including Divine Ayats' Fitra30 COVID-19 Protocol.

Divine Ayat's

Fitra30

COVID-19 PROTOCOL

(Patent Pending)

RNA viruses, COVID-19 in particular, are highly mutagenic- up to a million times higher than that of their hosts therefore, it is essential to build host resilience and defense mechanisms to ward off entry of this dis-ease into the body. The Fitra30 COVID-19 Protocol consists of natural treatments that stimulate and strengthen defense and healing mechanisms which are intrinsic to the host. These treatments are designed to specifically target COVID-19 by 1) blocking of pathways to SARS-CoV2 cellular entry and 2) Riding the body of COVID-19. Divine Ayats' Fitra30 COVID-19 Protocol is useful for individuals who desire effective natural treatments to prevent and treat COVID-19 as opposed to (or in conjunction with) vaccines and standard treatments. In Arabic the word "fitra" means "a state of purity and innocence". Muslims believe that all humans were born in this state or "natural disposition". Divine Ayats' Fitra30 COVID-19 Protocol is a 30-day program designed to guide participants back to a state of purity Spiritually, Physically, Mentally, and Emotionally.

This protocol consists of three features:

1) The Milhu Shamsi Herbal Formulation (MSHF). MSHF is designed to prevent and treat COVID-19 by targeting internal mechanisms which act as conduits for COVID-19 infection such as ICAM-1 and CCR5.

2) Induction of autophagy through herbal medicine and intermittent fasting. The term "autophagy" is Greek, meaning "eating of self". It is a sophisticated way by which the body rids itself of harmful pathogens (bacteria, viral particles, etc.) on a cellular level to restore homeostasis (87). In dis-ease recovery, autophagy can be thought as the body's desperate, self-destructive attempt at survival. Autophagy may in fact be the last immune defense against infectious pathogens that penetrate intracellularly (88). SARS-CoV-2 infection suppresses autophagy (89).

Interventions include Autophagy Jumpstart Herbal Blend (AJHB) and lifestyle modifications (i.e., intermittent fasting, proper diet, exercise, and sleep recommendations). A proven way of inducing autophagy is by food restriction (intermittent fasting), which upregulates autophagy in many organs (90).

Fasting plays an important role in Islamic Medicine. Once per year Muslims are obliged to participate in Ramadan in which they fast from sunrise to sundown. Outside of Ramadan, it is encouraged for Muslims to fast at least 11 days during the month, to include; Mondays, Thursdays, and the 13, 14, and 15th of each month (according to the Islamic Calendar). Eating in moderation outside of these times is encouraged and recommended foods include (but are not limited to) Prophetic Foods (i.e., honey- which contains strong antifungal properties against Candida albicans infection (91), grapes - which are high in antioxidant Resveratrol which helps to induce autophagy (92), and pomegranates- which suppresses necrosis (93).

3) Divine Ayat's Spiritual, Emotional, and Mental Rejuvenation Program (SEM-RP) . COVID-19 has greatly affected many lives around the world. The combination of uncertainty and quarantining is causing depression, anxiety, sleep problems, and psychological distress (94).

Divine Ayat's SMER Program is a 30-day guided meditation program designed to reduce stress. In a previous study, after 3 weeks of meditation students reported feeling less anxious, stressed, and displayed greater improvements in attentional control (95).

Funding

The author received no financial support for this research, authorship, and/or publication of this article.

Author Contributions

Taliah Safah Muhammad wrote the manuscript.

Declaration of Competing Interests

The author is the Owner of Divine Ayat, LLC. and patent holder of Divine Ayats' Fitra30 COVID-19 Protocol.

Acknowledgments

I thank Allah for entrusting me with the knowledge, skills, and abilities necessary to complete this work. May it be a benefit and guidance to all of mankind. Ameen.

Chapter Two

WHAT OUR HANDS HAVE EARNED

Allah, The Most High, says in The Qur'an;

ظَهَرَ ٱلْفَسَادُ فِى ٱلْبَرِّ وَٱلْبَحْرِ بِمَا كَسَبَتْ أَيْدِى ٱلنَّاسِ لِيُذِيقَهُم بَعْضَ ٱلَّذِى عَمِلُوا۟
لَعَلَّهُمْ يَرْجِعُونَ

"Evil (sins and disobedience to Allah) has appeared on land and sea because of what the hands of men have earned (by oppression and evil deeds), that He (Allah) may make them taste a part of that which they have done, in order that they may return (by repenting to Allah, and begging His Pardon).

Surah Ar-Rum, 30:41

The Widespread Sins

We live in a time where sin has become widespread and, in many cases, deemed acceptable by the masses. One such sin is that of homosexuality which is a deviant way that takes one far away from the path of Allah, The Most High. The caller to this path is none other than Shaytan (Satan), the enemy of mankind, whereby he seduces the servant into desiring for him or herself that which Allah, The Exalted, has made impermissible. Other widespread sins of this generation include the acceptance of transgender identities whereby men can dress like women and be referred to as "she", "it", or "they". Conversely, women who choose this lifestyle don the clothing and mannerisms of men and may request to be referred to as "he", "it", or "they". Hormone therapy is another widespread evil through which young women and girls can take testosterone pills or boys and men can take estrogen supplements in order change their features to that of the opposite sex. Some of these Western medicines are so potent that a male can become undistinguishable from a female once he completes treatment as his features, voice, and even mannerisms are completely that of a woman! I have even read a story where a man upon this unfortunate affair tricked another man into marrying him. The latter has yet to discover he has married a man and does not understand why his wife has yet to become pregnant! SubhanAllah. May Allah, The Most Kind, protect our sons and daughters from these and all other deceptions, Ameen.

Further, many of these people proceed deeper into misguidance and elect to have sexual reassignment surgeries, whereby they pay a devilish doctor to cut their private parts into the shapes of the opposite sex. These acts constitute complete disbelief in Allah, The Most Wise, as it is:

1. A rejection of Allah's Infinite Wisdom-

Every person was destined to be here on earth in the generation that Allah, The Most High, decreed. Human creation is not a spontaneous event that resulted from animal evolution or the wild notions of "random natural selection". Further, Allah, The Most Wise, did not make a mistake when assigning genders or any other matter regarding the human race. In fact, everything that would come into existence, be it humans, animals, plants, our deeds, etc., was decreed by

Allah, The Most High, 50,000 years before he created the heavens and the earth. Finally, our creation is above that of other creations (i.e., the animals, jinn, etc.) and so, we should not attempt to imitate or align with their creations in any way. There are many persons who will try to justify homosexuality by pointing to various instances in nature. These people lack understanding and knowledge of why man was created and the position Allah, The Most Wise, gave him (mankind) over all other creations in the earth.

Abdullah reported that Umm Habiba رَحِمَهُ ٱللَّٰه, the wife of Allah's Apostle (ﷺ), said:

Allah, enable me to derive benefit from my husband, the Messenger of Allah (ﷺ), and from my father Abu Sufyan and from my brother Mu'awiya. Allah's Apostle (ﷺ) said: You have asked from Allah about durations of life already set, and the length of days already allotted and the sustenance the share of which has been fixed. Allah would not do anything earlier before its due time, or He would not delay anything beyond its due time. And if you were to ask Allah to provide you refuge from the torment of the Hell Fire, or from the torment of the grave, it would have good in store for you and better for you also. He (the narrator) further said: Mention was made before him about monkeys, and Mis'ar (one of the narrators) said: I think that (the narrator) also (made a mention) of the swine, which had suffered metamorphosis. Thereupon he (the Holy Prophet) said: Verily, Allah did not cause the race of those which suffered metamorphosis to grow or they were not survived by young ones. Monkeys and swine had been in existence even before (the metamorphosis of the human beings).

Sahih Muslim, Book 46, Hadith 49

Abdullah b. 'Amr b. al-'As رَحِمَهُ ٱللَّٰه reported:

I heard Allah's Messenger (ﷺ) as saying: Allah ordained the measures (of quality) of the creation fifty thousand years before He created the heavens and the earth, as His Throne was upon water.

Sahih Muslim, Book 46, Hadith 27

<u>Allah, The Exalted, says in The Qur'an:</u>

لَقَدْ خَلَقْنَا ٱلْإِنسَٰنَ فِىٓ أَحْسَنِ تَقْوِيمٍ

"Verily, We created man in the best stature (mould).

Surah At-Tin, 95:4

2. Complete ungratefulness to Allah, The Most Kind –

Our bodies are a loan to us from Allah, The Exalted. Desecration of this vessel through doing acts of disobedience (i.e., not worshipping Allah and oppressing one's body through sexual deviance and other sins) is all ungratefulness to Allah.

<u>Allah, The Exalted, says in The Qur'an:</u>

وَإِذْ تَأَذَّنَ رَبُّكُمْ لَئِن شَكَرْتُمْ لَأَزِيدَنَّكُمْ ۖ وَلَئِن كَفَرْتُمْ إِنَّ عَذَابِى لَشَدِيدٌ

"And (remember) when your Lord proclaimed: "If you give thanks (by accepting Faith and worshipping none but Allah), I will give you more (of My Blessings); but if you are thankless (i.e. disbelievers), verily My punishment is indeed severe."

Surah Ibrahim, 14:7

3. <u>A means for total alignment with Shaytan and his people.</u>

Those who have aligned with Shaytan through participation in sexual deviancy be it actively or passively are guilty of the promotion of evil on earth. This alignment, the stronger it becomes, will ultimately lead to the degradation of the society through the disruption of health, the family unit, and ultimately the cycle of reproduction.

<u>Allah, The Exalted, says in The Qur'an:</u>

لَآ إِكْرَاهَ فِى ٱلدِّينِ ۖ قَد تَّبَيَّنَ ٱلرُّشْدُ مِنَ ٱلْغَىِّ ۚ فَمَن يَكْفُرْ بِٱلطَّٰغُوتِ وَيُؤْمِنۢ بِٱللَّهِ فَقَدِ
ٱسْتَمْسَكَ بِٱلْعُرْوَةِ ٱلْوُثْقَىٰ لَا ٱنفِصَامَ لَهَا ۗ وَٱللَّهُ سَمِيعٌ عَلِيمٌ

ٱللَّهُ وَلِىُّ ٱلَّذِينَ ءَامَنُوا۟ يُخْرِجُهُم مِّنَ ٱلظُّلُمَٰتِ إِلَى ٱلنُّورِ ۖ وَٱلَّذِينَ كَفَرُوٓا۟ أَوْلِيَآؤُهُمُ
ٱلطَّٰغُوتُ يُخْرِجُونَهُم مِّنَ ٱلنُّورِ إِلَى ٱلظُّلُمَٰتِ ۗ أُو۟لَٰٓئِكَ أَصْحَٰبُ ٱلنَّارِ ۖ هُمْ فِيهَا خَٰلِدُونَ

"There is no compulsion in religion. Verily, the Right Path has become distinct from the wrong path. Whoever disbelieves in Taghut and believes in Allah, then he has grasped the most trustworthy handhold that will never break. And Allah is All-Hearer, All-Knower. Allah is the Wali (Protector or Guardian) of those who believe. He brings them out from darkness into light. But as for those who disbelieve, their Auliya' (supporters and helpers) are Taghut [false deities and false leaders], they bring them out from light into darkness. Those are the dwellers of the Fire, and they will abide therein forever."

Surah Al-Baqarah, 2:256-257

<u>The Physical Manifestations of Sin</u>

In Islamic Medicine, there is no separation between religion and science. For every spiritual transgression, there are physical phenomena to which it relates. This cause-and-effect relationship between sins and mortality can be evidenced in the Qur'an when Allah, The Exalted, says;

أَفَأَمِنَ ٱلَّذِينَ مَكَرُوا ٱلسَّيِّـَٔاتِ أَن يَخْسِفَ ٱللَّهُ بِهِمُ ٱلْأَرْضَ أَوْ يَأْتِيَهُمُ ٱلْعَذَابُ مِنْ حَيْثُ لَا يَشْعُرُونَ

أَوْ يَأْخُذَهُمْ فِى تَقَلُّبِهِمْ فَمَا هُم بِمُعْجِزِينَ

أَوْ يَأْخُذَهُمْ عَلَىٰ تَخَوُّفٍ فَإِنَّ رَبَّكُمْ لَرَءُوفٌ رَّحِيمٌ

"Do then those who devise evil plots feel secure (immune) that Allah will not sink them into the earth, or that the torment will not seize them from directions they perceive not? Or that He may catch them in the midst of their going to and fro (in their jobs), so that there be no escape for them (from Allah's punishment)? Or that He may catch them with gradual wasting (of their wealth and health)? Truly! Your Lord is indeed full of Kindness, Most Merciful.

Surah An-Nahl, 16:45-47

COVID-19 is upon us as a consequence for our sins and, moreover, it serves to warn us of our spiritual misdeeds. Not only has most of the world decriminalized homosexuality, but it has also given legal protections and rights to those who practice these acts. According to Pew Research data, 30 countries around the world have legalized gay marriage in the last eleven years, including; Mexico (2009), The Netherlands (2000), Belgium (2003), Canada (2005), Spain (2005), South Africa (2006), Norway (2008), Sweden (2009), Iceland (2010), Portugal (2010), Argentina (2010), Denmark (2012), Uruguay (2013), New Zealand (2013), France (2013), Brazil (2013), England and Wales (2013), Scotland (2014), Luxembourg (2014), Finland (2015), Ireland (2015), Greenland (2015), United States (2015), Columbia (2016), Germany (2017), Malta (2017), Australia (2017), Austria (2019), Taiwan (2019), Ecuador (2019), Northern Ireland (2019), Costa Rica (2020) (1). It is unfortunate that those who speak out against this deviancy are deemed; "homophobic", "unaccepting", "judgmental", and some dare to say "ungodly"! Sexual deviance has permeated so deeply within society that not even the babies and youth are immune from this dis-ease. Many misguided parents have the idea that they will allow their child to choose his or her gender once they (the young child) are ready. Until this time, they deem the child as "non-binary", meaning, they have no specified gender. This is a great injustice committed against innocent children.

Abu Huraira رحمة الله reported Allah's Messenger (ﷺ) as saying:

No child is born but upon Fitra (Islam). He then said. Recite: The nature made by Allah in which He created man, there is no altering of Allah's nature; that is the right religion. "

Sahih Muslim, Book 46, Hadith 36

In another narration by Abu Huraira رحمة الله:

Allah's Messenger (ﷺ) said, "No child is born except on Al-Fitra (Islam) and then his parents make him Jewish, Christian or Magian, as an animal produces a perfect young animal: do you see any part of its body amputated? " Then he recited; 'The religion of pure Islamic Faith (Hanifa), (i.e., to worship none but Allah), The pure Islamic nature with which He (Allah) has created mankind. Let there be no change in Allah's religion (i.e., to join none in Allah's worship). That is the straight religion; but most of men know not ... " (30.30)

Sahih al-Bukhari, Book 65, Hadith 297

Sexual Deviancy: Lessons from the Past

Homosexuality first appeared in the earth with the people of Prophet Lut عَلَيْهِ ٱلسَّلَامُ. Allah, The Most High, says in The Qur'an;

وَلُوطًا إِذْ قَالَ لِقَوْمِهِۦٓ أَتَأْتُونَ ٱلْفَـٰحِشَةَ مَا سَبَقَكُم بِهَا مِنْ أَحَدٍ مِّنَ ٱلْعَـٰلَمِينَ

إِنَّكُمْ لَتَأْتُونَ ٱلرِّجَالَ شَهْوَةً مِّن دُونِ ٱلنِّسَآءِ ۚ بَلْ أَنتُمْ قَوْمٌ مُّسْرِفُونَ

وَمَا كَانَ جَوَابَ قَوْمِهِۦٓ إِلَّآ أَن قَالُوٓا۟ أَخْرِجُوهُم مِّن قَرْيَتِكُمْ ۖ إِنَّهُمْ أُنَاسٌ يَتَطَهَّرُونَ

"And (remember) Lut (Lot), when he said to his people: "Do you commit the worst sin such as none preceding you has committed in the *Alamin* (mankind and jinn)? Verily, you practice your lusts on men instead of women. Nay, but you are a people transgressing beyond bounds (by committing great sins). And the answer of his people was only that they said: "Drive them out of your town, these are indeed men who want to be pure (from sins)!"

Surah Al-A'raf, 7:80-82

Prophet Lut عَلَيْهِ ٱلسَّلَامُ spent many years warning his people yet they turned away and were persistent in the wrongdoing. Due to their persistence in wrongdoing and failure to take heed of the warnings of Allah, the Most High, they were ultimately destroyed;

كَذَّبَتْ قَوْمُ لُوطٍۭ بِٱلنُّذُرِ

إِنَّآ أَرْسَلْنَا عَلَيْهِمْ حَاصِبًا إِلَّآ ءَالَ لُوطٍ ۖ نَّجَّيْنَـٰهُم بِسَحَرٍ

نِّعْمَةً مِّنْ عِندِنَا ۚ كَذَٰلِكَ نَجْزِى مَن شَكَرَ

"The people of Lut (Lot) denied the warnings. Verily, We sent against them a violent storm of stones (which destroyed them all) except the family of Lut (Lot), We saved them in the last hour of the night. As a Favor from Us. Thus do We reward him who gives thanks (by obeying Us)."

Surah Al-Qamar, 54:33-35

It is important to remember here, that not all of Prophet Lut's عَلَيْهِ ٱلسَّلَامُ family members were saved as Allah, The Most High, says in The Qur'an:

إِلَّآ ءَالَ لُوطٍ إِنَّا لَمُنَجُّوهُمْ أَجْمَعِينَ
إِلَّا ٱمْرَأَتَهُۥ قَدَّرْنَآ ۙ إِنَّهَا لَمِنَ ٱلْغَٰبِرِينَ

"(All) except the family of Lut (Lot). Them all we are surely going to save (from destruction). Except his wife, of whom We have decreed that she shall be of those who remain behind (i.e., she will be destroyed).

Surah Al-Hijr, 15:59-60

Prophet Lut's عَلَيْهِ ٱلسَّلَامُ wife did not forbid wrongdoing (homosexuality) by joining her husband's call. Instead, she helped the homosexuals against her husband and facilitated a way for them to carry out their lusts! She was so engrossed in her life with the people that her heart had become intertwined with them, so much so, she was destined to be destroyed along with them.

How many of us Muslim are like the wife of Prophet Lut عَلَيْهِ ٱلسَّلَامُ? It is shameful to say that in this time there are many

Muslims who are helpers and supporters of these people despite their (the Muslims) prayers and fasting. They support western political systems by voting and, even worse, they often align the parties that support the practice of homosexuality throughout the world such as the liberalists in America. They keep silent on their jobs and within their families, choosing not to warn the homosexual persons around them of the consequences of their sins. They protest in the streets (which is something forbidden in Islam), offering solidarity and support to the corrupters of the earth! These Muslims think they are upon something good, but in truth, their abstinence from homosexual acts means nothing if they actively support the systems, organizations, and persons who promote it.

Sexual Deviance: An Analysis of Current Affairs

According to a 2021 report, The United States of America remains the most powerful country in the world (2). Respected and often mimicked by other nations, the U.S. has significant influence on societies around the globe. In 2015, the U.S. Supreme Court declared the ban on gay marriage unconstitutional, defiantly rejecting Allah's Divine Laws regarding marriage. Since that time, there has been a sharp increase Sexually Transmitted Disease (STDs). According to a press release by the U.S. Centers for Disease Control (CDC) there has been close to a 30% increase in cases of chlamydia, gonorrhea, and syphilis from 2015 to 2019. According to Raul Romaguera, DMD, MPH, acting director for the CDC's Division of STD Prevention; "Less than 20 years ago, gonorrhea rates in the U.S. were at historic lows, syphilis was close to elimination, and advances in chlamydia diagnostics made it easier to detect infections…that progress has since unraveled, and our STD defenses are down. We must prioritize and focus our efforts to regain this lost ground and control the spread of STDs." This report also noted that the rate of STD infection is 5-8 times higher for African Americans / Blacks than White or Hispanic persons (3).

Out of all the STD's identified, the cases of syphilis had the sharpest increase, rising 71% between 2014-2018. In this same time period, cases gonorrhea and chlamydia had 63% and 19% rate increases, respectively. It was found that gay and bisexual men make up nearly 50% of all 2019 Primary and Secondary (P&S) syphilis cases. Further, 42% of all MSM (men who sleep with men) with P&S syphilis were known to be living with diagnosed HIV. Congenial Syphilis has also seen a startling 185% increase in the rate of infection in the U.S. Congenial Syphilis occurs when a pregnant woman who is infected with syphilis transmits the disease to her unborn child (4). Historically it has been documented that untreated syphilis in pregnant women, if acquired four years before delivery, can lead to infection in the unborn child in up to 80% of all cases. Stillborn infant death is another serious complication occurring in up to 40% of all cases (5).

Syphilis is caused by the bacterium Treponema pallidum. Currently, there is only one antibiotic believed to effectively treat syphilis in pregnant women and newborns however, there is a severe shortage. When left untreated, syphilis can increase the likelihood of HIV transmission and infection. Complications of Congenial Syphilis include meningitis, anemia, bone abnormalities, and other physical, and neurological disabilities in infants (5).

From Sexual Deviance to Marriage: Why Eugenicists Are Upset

Historically, the complications of untreated syphilis in the U.S. have mainly affected African Americans and Hispanics. However, the rise in the numbers of interracial cohabitation (dating), interracial marriage, and bisexual identification, makes syphilis and other untreated STDs a growing threat to the health and fertility of all races particularly Whites and Asians. This phenomenon has much to do with *who* these two groups are dating and marrying.

According to a 2013 report, Asian Americans are the fastest growing racial group in the U.S surpassing Hispanics (6). The U.S. has seen more than a five-fold increase in interracial marriage since it was legalized in 1967 by the U.S. Supreme Court in the landmark case of Loving vs. Virginia. As of 2019, one-in-six newlyweds in the U.S. were married to someone of a different race. Asian and Hispanic newlyweds were found to be the most likely of all races to intermarry – with Asians being 29% more likely while Hispanics are 27% more likely to marry someone of a different race. This amount increases for U.S. born Asians and Hispanics to 46% and 39%, respectively. The largest share of intermarried couples includes one Hispanic and one White spouse which accounts for 46% of all interracial marriages. The second largest group consists of one Black or Multiracial spouse and one White spouse, accounting for 23% of all interracial marriages. One Asian spouse and one White spouse accounts for 15% of all interracial marriages in the U.S. It is important to note here that has been found that black men are twice as likely than black women to marry outside of their race.

Additionally, the intermarriage rate has tripled for Black Americans since the 1980s. Further, Asian women are more likely than Asian men to marry outside of their race (7). Interracial marriage in has naturally led to a rise in multiracial and multiethnic babies. In 2015, one-in-seven U.S. infants were multiracial / multiethnic, tripling the amount from 1980 (8).

A 2017 study found that among U.S. cohabitors 18% have a partner of a different race or ethnicity. While whites were the least likely to cohabit with someone of a different race (12%) - Blacks (20%), Hispanics (24%), and Asians (46%) topped the charts. These trends in interracial dating can be attributed to the more liberal, higher educated (secular), and forward-thinking members of the Millennial and Generation X populations (9).

A 2021 Gallop Poll found that 5.6% of Americans identify as Lesbian, Gay, Bisexual, or Transgender (LGBT). This is a significant increase from 4.5% in 2017. Further, this poll found that 56% of all LGBT people identify as bisexual (10) meaning they desire men and women equally. It is important to remember that this data does not accurately reflect the number people practicing bisexual lifestyles. As a 2019 Pew Research report revealed that bisexual men are 26% less likely than gay men and lesbians to disclose their sexual preferences to the people in their lives (11).

When You Violate God's Laws, Your Enemy Will Violate You: A Notable Violation of Informed Consent:

The U.S. Government owes much of its scientific insights about the complications of untreated syphilis to the involuntary sacrifice of African Americans. In 1932, The Public Health Service in conjunction with Tuskegee Institute began a study entitled; "Tuskegee Study of Untreated Syphilis in the Negro Male." The study enrolled 600 participants- 399 with syphilis, and 201 free from the dis-ease. The group with syphilis were never told they were infected, and all participants thought they were being evaluated for "bad blood" which during that time was thought to include syphilis, anemia, and fatigue. The participants were offered free medical exams, meals, and burial stipends in exchange for their consent and involvement. These generous stipends were welcomed as the Great Depression had hit the South hard. Despite the outward appeal of the study, it had two fundamental problems. Firstly, the participants were never truly informed of the goals of the study. Remember, the infected patients were completely unaware of their status. Secondly, the study was only intended to last for six months but instead went on for 40 years, until 1972.

The scientists and doctors involved with the study decided to follow each participant until death in order to record how the dis-ease affected their health and the health of their families. In 1947, penicillin became a viable and effective option for treating syphilis. Unfortunately, the participants of the study were never offered this treatment. Nearly 100 participants would die from untreated syphilis and the individual effects this dis-ease had on their wives and children's health remains unknown to this day. In 1972, an Associated Press article alerted the public and ultimately the U.S. Government to investigate the ethics of the study. Congress would ultimately decide that the participants of the study were deceived, as they were not given the facts needed to give a valid informed consent. The study ended in that same year and in 1973 Congress held a class-action lawsuit on behalf of the participants. In 1974, a $10 million dollar settlement was reached and on May 16, 1997 President Bill Clinton apologized to the participants on behalf of the U.S. Government (12).

It is important to note that the U.S. Public Health Service is still in operation today. Functioning as a division of The U.S. Department of Health & Human Services, The Public Health Service oversees ten governmental components that are essential to public health in the U.S. and abroad. To date, the components running under the Public Health Service include; the Agency for Healthcare Research and Quality (AHRQ), Agency for Toxic Substances and Disease Registry (ATSDR), the Centers for Disease Control and Prevention (CDC), the Food and Drug Administration (FDA), Health Resources and Services Administration (HRSA), Indian Health Service (HIS), National

Institutes of Health (NIH), Substance Abuse and Mental Health Services (SAMHSA), Office of the Assistant Secretary for Planning and Evaluation (ASPE), Office of Global Affairs (OGA) (13).

Changing Natures

Allah, The All Wise, has allowed this trial of COVID-19 to fall upon us because we as a human race have turned away from His Divine Laws. We have had many warnings to turn back from our sins and repent, yet most people on earth remain heedless to Allah's Call. We have striven hard to superficially change our nature through transgenderism, hormone therapies, and sexual reassignment surgeries that as a consequence, Allah, The Most Wise, has allowed an enemy who has been working diligently to change our nature at its most fundamental point- *our DNA,* to have their way.

This enemy has never operated with dignity or ethics for that matter. They are relentless in their pursuit to reach their goals and due to our collective turning away from Allah, The Most High, we are now faced with new dis-eases and challenges that our forefathers never suffered. These are sure signs that Allah, The Most High, is not pleased with us. Though we have an enemy indeed, we can blame only ourselves for this affliction. We are most certainly reaping the harvest of what our hands have collectively earned. However, there still lies the opportunity for immense blessings to descend upon us if we but humble ourselves, acknowledge our faults, and turn to Allah, The Most

High, in repentance and servitude. For Allah is Al-Gafoor, The One Who Forgives again and again. May Allah, The Most High, make us of those who take heed and mend our conduct. Ameen.

May He, The Most High, also keep us far away from being among those who on The Day of Judgement will say;

وَقَالُوا لَوْ كُنَّا نَسْمَعُ أَوْ نَعْقِلُ مَا كُنَّا فِيٓ أَصْحَـٰبِ ٱلسَّعِيرِ

"…had we but listened or used our intelligence, we would not have been among the dwellers of the blazing Fire."

Surah Al-Mulk, 63:10

Ameen.

Chapter Three

THE MAKINGS OF A CULT

Eugenics & The Survival of the Fittest

Eugenics (yoo-JEH-niks):

A biological and social science movement which promotes and facilitates the use of practices such as selective breeding designed at improving the genetic composition of a society (1).

For thousands of years mankind has practiced some form of eugenics. Greek philosopher Plato peddled the idea of "selective mating" to Greek government officials. He believed that this type of mating would aid in the development of "guardian" characteristics in the offspring of those who were paired. Plato's unrestrained imagination led him to create a fictional tripartite society consisting of, producers, auxiliaries, and guardians. Guardians, he fathomed, should be those responsible for ruling the city (2).

In the Spartan era, each child was inspected by a group of elders called the Gerousia. This council was comprised of men over the age of 60 who had the responsibility to determine if the child was fit to live or die. The council might deem a child unfit to live due to physical or mental imperfection and thus sentenced to death by being thrown from the summit of Mount Taygetus. The Spartan practice of eugenics did not stop with the murder of innocent children. Starting at age seven girls and boys were adopted by the state and raised in camps. There they were indoctrinated with oppressive

Spartan beliefs and physically trained with much vigor to carry out their assigned roles within society. Further, at the age of 21, males were placed in army units and as a part of their training they hunted the innocent "helots"- neighboring citizens who had been conquered by the Spartans. What is interesting is that in its prime, it is believed that Sparta consisted of around 9,000 citizens who ruled over at least 100,000 helots (3). In Sparta, and many times throughout history, the ruling group was significantly outnumbered.

In the Roman Republic, where the religious authorities were apathetic to personal beliefs or privately funded cults, eugenics was enforced by the government but implemented by the family. If a child were deemed "unfit to live" it would be the duty of the father to kill his child immediately (4).

Though eugenics as a concept has been practiced throughout many millennia, the name of this movement was only coined at the turn of the 19th the century by Sir Francis Galton. Galton believed that desirable human traits are attributed to genes, and how those genes are passed down from parent to child. These ideas became appealing to Galton after reading his half-cousin Chares Darwin's work entitled; "On the Origin of Species" which was published in 1859.

In his book, Darwin asserts many fallacious beliefs including the belief that that mankind originated from apes. A naturalist who spent much of his time traveling and study animals and plants, Darwin sought to apply his perceptions about their development to humans. During childhood, he learned that breeders would often select the best animals to mate in an effort to produce desirable herds. He decided that "nature" must also do the same thing and he called this concept "natural selection".

Darwin theorized that mutations in each generation of a particular species coupled with changes in environmental conditions could make one group from that species more likely to win the competition for scarce food which would ensure their ability to reproduce. If we apply this theory to humans, as it was intended to be applied, it would state; *in the presence of genetic mutations, if a condition in the environment (i.e., the natural world) were changed, the race that has more biological ability to adapt would be the ones to survive.*

Other factors that would further ensure their survival would include access and control over the food supply as well as ownership of environments that are conducive to human reproduction (i.e. land, housing, clean water, fresh air, etc.). Further, the races who are not able to biologically adapt to this change in the environment would inevitably become sick – many dying from biological deficiencies and environmental factors while many others would die from starvation. *Ultimately, these "less fit" races would be eliminated due to their inability to maintain an environment that is conducive to human reproduction.*

This theory seemed to be fueled by not only observation, but also with Darwin's agreement with the predictions of an English economist named Thomas Malthus. In his work entitled; "An Essay on the Principle of Population", Malthus asserted that the human population would one day grow faster than the food supply. Consequently, the overpopulation of humans would lead to famine ushering in the times of the "survival of the fittest". Darwin further concluded that hereditary information is stored within an organism and its identification would be essential in further explaining and exploiting his theories of natural selection (5).

Galton would echo his cousins' ideas and would ultimately take them many steps further by establishing the science of Eugenics. Despite him being a small-minded European racist, Galton was educated, well connected, articulate, and thus able to promote his large volume of distorted, deviant, and devilish themes to audiences who actually listened. On May 16, 1904, Galton presented before the Sociological Society at a meeting in the School of Economics at London University. At this meeting, his thoughts were on full display. While reading his speech, I imagined Galton standing from a tall and mighty pulpit, holding a fabricated holy book, delivering his verdicts while gazing down upon mankind from on high. Had he lived thousands of years ago in Rome, he most certainly would have been one of those who thought the development of a guardian class a moral obligation.

During his speech, Galton said as much when he declared that one group, not the masses, should decide what is best for all of humanity. He argued that if every species were able to contribute to the discussion of what is best for humanity there would most certainly be much bickering due to the variations in the species, their lifestyles, and the specific needs of each group. This great differing, he believed, would make reaching an agreement about what is best for the society as whole impossible. As any great authoritarian would, Galton offered what he believed to be essential principles that every creature would agree to. These principles centered around the ideas that; 1) physical fitness is better than ill health; 2) hardiness is better than defect; 3) humans would rather be prepared for their roles in life as opposed to unprepared and; 4) all humans would rather be represented by the "best specimens" of their kind as opposed to the worst.

To cater to what he supposed every human would want if given a choice, Galton proceeded to set forth goals for Eugenics. The first goal was to see that each class would be represented by its best specimens or members as once that is established, these groups could be left alone to develop their own civilizations according to their own ways. The second goal included calling for a "meeting of the minds" by bringing together influential persons from each class, then employing them in roles so they can contribute to the advancements of the next generation.

Like a well-planned con man, Galton seemed to have all the answers. In the next part of his speech, he spelled out how Eugenicists might achieve their new goals. Galton recommended that the elitist members of society (i.e., the wealthy, intelligent, scholarly, and biologically well-suited, etc.) be actively engaged in the science of heredity. Not only did he propose heredity be studied and quantified, but he also championed the dissemination of that knowledge throughout the community of

Eugenicists, this way, everyone in their global network might have access to it. It was at this point that he took up the flag where his cousin Darwin left off.

Galton ascertained that civilized nations of the past monitored the fertility and reproduction rates of the upper class. Accordingly, he believed, these civilizations should be studied in-depth, and their methods adopted. In addition to the study of fertility and reproduction, he also encouraged the study of relationships and marriage. Based upon his preliminary observations on these subjects, Galton discovered that few species would be able to maintain fertility when "their liberty is restricted and their struggles for livelihood abolished". However, the ones that do survive are often the fittest, most productive, and have more capability of creating or adapting to a new, more civilized society.

His next observation would serve as a compass, guiding Eugenicists of the future towards the purpose, focus, and "therapeutic target" of their genetic research for years to come. Galton expressed that while the fittest would thrive, procreate, and civilize under harsh conditions, there would be one race that would also continue to exist and remain fertile, though, they would be far from civilized. That race, he believed, was the *negro*. This statement would leave Eugenicists of the future with a looming question, *if the negro survives and procreates despite harsh conditions, what do we do with them?* Today's Eugenicists have determined the answer is *extermination*, but we will discuss that more later.

Further, Galton encouraged historians to write biographies about successful Eugenicists to familiarize the public with the subject. He also encouraged the study of social influences affecting marriage. His last words during this address are perhaps the most telling. Galton encouraged Eugenicists to swiftly take up the work that he meticulously outlined. He encouraged them to be persistent and relentless in making eugenics an important academic inquiry until it is accepted as fact through genetic research. Galton ended his speech by saying;

"It (eugenics) must be introduced into the national conscience, like a new religion. It has, indeed, strong claims to become an orthodox religious, tenet of the future, for eugenics co-operate with the workings of nature by securing that humanity shall be represented by the fittest races. What nature does blindly, slowly, and ruthlessly, man may do providently, quickly, and kindly. As it lies within his power, so it becomes his duty to work in that direction. The improvement of our stock seems to me one of the highest objects that we can reasonably attempt. We are ignorant of the ultimate destinies of humanity, but feel perfectly sure that it is as noble a work to raise its level, in the sense already explained, as it would be disgraceful to abase it. I see no impossibility in eugenics becoming a religious dogma among mankind, but its details must first be worked out sedulously in the study. Overzeal leading to hasty action would do harm, by holding out expectations of a near golden age, which will certainly be falsified and cause the science to be discredited. The first and main point is to secure the general intellectual acceptance of

eugenics as a hopeful and most important study. Then let its principles work into the heart of the nation, which will gradually give practical effect to them in ways that we may not wholly foresee." (5)

In one speech, Galton had become the faux Prophet and Messenger of the Modern Eugenics Movement. His Holy books included ancient scrolls from fallen civilizations and the speculative writings of those greedy for the life of this world and its ownership. He would take his direction from his nafs (lower soul) that was polluted with the racist biases lurking in his heart and mind. Believing himself to be well equipped, he would call forth to those like him, possessing comparable intellect, and would instruct them to research, write, and ultimately subdue the world.

Chapter Four

THEY STROVE, THEY ACHIEVED

The Devotees of Eugenics

Fellow Eugenicists in every sector promptly heeded to Galton's call. Using their influence and position they vehemently thrust their beliefs upon society both domestically and internationally. Eugenicists penetrated the realms of academics, religion, politics, social and civic organizations, science, and medicine. The ideologies they pushed greatly appealed to the hearts of middle and upper-class members of almost every race throughout the world.

Eugenics in Education

Eugenics became a popular subject taught in universities in the early 1900s. By 1914, over 40 U.S. colleges and universities offered courses in Eugenics including the University of Richmond, New York University, and The University of Florida (1-2). In normal fashion, blacks would follow whites due to their misguided quest for equality in America. In 1912, Howard University would offer a variety of Eugenics courses taught by Thomas Wyatt Turner. Turners' views on Eugenics deviated from the norm in that he believed black hereditary issues came primarily from poor environmental conditions and low education, though he did agree genes played a role as well. His version of "black eugenics" would ultimately align back with Galton's version of Eugenics, in that Turner believed that the black middle class should be the group to represent and lead the black race while setting the standards for civilization to its lower-class members (3).

Elsewhere in black academia, W.E.B. Du Bois, a Black sociologist, was arguing the same. A graduate of the historically black Fisk University, Du Bois published a eugenicist themed work of sorts entitled; "The Talented Tenth". In his book, he argued that the talented tenth were the "exception" from "the mass of ignorant Negroes". He proposed that this small group of exceptional black men would be the ones to save the race. He believed that education was the key factor in the development of "good stock"(4). He also voiced that most negros were unfit to be parents and though he opposed institutionalized sterilization, he endorsed abortion in the black community as a form of birth control (5). His position would echo that of his white peers, namely Margret Sanger, a proud feminist and Eugenicist, and the founder of the U.S. birth control movement which deliberately targeted inner-city blacks (6).

Eugenics in Social & Civic Organizations

Due to the penetration of eugenicist mindsets in black academia, Greek Fraternities and Sororities began to appear. Just like their white counterparts, Greek organizations would act as a type of secrete society providing a hierarchal structure aimed at dividing members of their race based upon education and other socioeconomic factors. The first of those organizations was Alpha Phi Alpha which was formed on the campus of Cornell University in 1906 of which W.E.B. Du Bois is a celebrated member. Meanwhile, the true leaders within the Eugenics cult were forming more far-reaching organizations to promote their beliefs of genetic white supremacy and to solicit support and funding. Some of these organizations included the

British Eugenics Education Society in 1907 and The American Eugenics Society of 1921. To fortify their efforts, Eugenicists internationally organized through the International Federation of Eugenics Organizations which was founded in London in 1912.

Eugenics in Religion

Christian churches played a major role in garnering public support and ultimately swaying popular opinion about Eugenics. In 1921, the Roman Catholic Church endorsed the International Eugenics Conference. These conferences, which were held in London in 1921 and New York in 1921 and 1932, allowed Eugenicist all around the world to meet, propagate their beliefs, and develop methodologies that would pave the way for future Eugenicists.

In the black community, church leaders were used to support and enforce the Eugenicists population control plan for the negro. In 1939, Margret Sanger penned a letter to her friend Clarence Gamble, heir to the Proctor and Gamble fortune and private funder of abortion clinics. In the letter, Sanger laid out her plan to use the black church to influence the black communities' views on her racist endeavors.

"We do not want word to go out that we want to exterminate the Negro population, and the minister is the man who can straighten out that idea if it ever occurs to any of their more rebellious members," she wrote.

When accepting the Planned Parenthood's Margaret Sanger Award in Human Rights in 1969, Martin Luther King,

Jr., a popular black minister in U.S. history, would praise Sanger's "commitment" to the black community (7).

Sanger also received support from the Woman's Christian Temperance Union as they would prove effective in lobbying for government intervention in healthcare via eugenics reform in the U.S. and Canada (8).

Eugenics in Politics

Major progress was being made in the political arena as well. The rise in Chinese and Japanese immigrants in the early 1900s fueled existing xenophobia in the U.S. By 1913, 30 U.S. states had new anti-miscegenation laws which prevented the marriage of Whites to Native Americans and Asians (9). These types of laws had already been in existence as it pertains to Whites and Blacks since 1619.

Xenophobia towards Asians can be traced to the "yellow peril" ideology. This ideology is rooted in the same racist themes that have been used to minimalized black people throughout American history. It asserts that Asians or "yellow" people originate from apes and are barbaric, evil, mystical, rapists whom white society should be protected from (10). Throughout history, these perceptions would be promoted and enforced by law in the U.S., Russia, Germany, Canada, and Australia even prior to the Eugenics cult formation. However, the European bias towards Asians and Blacks gained new fervor as the Eugenicist ideology penetrated the world.

Eugenicists would promote the "yellow peril" themes through fictional and non-fictional literature and cinema. Two popular non-fiction works that gained worldwide attention were; "The Passing of the Great Race" by an American lawyer named Madison Grant in 1916 and "The Rising Tide of Color: The Threat Against White World Supremacy" by Lothrop Stoddard in 1920. In his work, Lothrop warned that white supremacy around the world was under a threat due to the population growth, rising nationalism, and industrialization in communities and nations of "people of color". It must be noted that Lothrop was an influential member of Margret B. Sangers American Birth Control League.

In cinema, novels, and comic books, Asian men were depicted as rapists who were after precious White women. Asian women, on the other hand, were often depicted as cunning prostitutes (11-13). All these efforts were done to deter race-mixing with Asians and to stoke the existing fears and insecurities of Europeans everywhere.

These attitudes would trickle down to the black community as many blacks would promote demeaning jokes about the size of Asian men's private parts which deterred black women from seeing them as potential mates. These acts all fall under "rumor mongering" and slander as many of these statements are vicious lies that were used as a means to browbeat and berate Asians. In Islam, these acts are strictly forbidden due to their ability to severely harm the victim.

Abdullah ibn Mas'ud رحمة الله reported: We were sitting with the Prophet, peace and blessings be upon him, when a man stood to leave, then another man spoke badly about him after he left. The Prophet said, "Pick your teeth." The man said, "O Messenger of Allah, why should I pick my teeth when I have not eaten meat?" The Prophet said, "You have eaten the flesh of your brother."

Source: al-Mu'jam al-Kabīr 9951

Just as the harm is great for the sin of slander, so is the punishment.

Hudhayfah رَحِمَهُ ٱللَّٰه reported: The Prophet, peace and blessings be upon him, said, "**The talebearer will not enter Paradise.**"

Sahīh al-Bukhārī 5709, Sahīh Muslim 105

This deliberate slander campaign by Eugenicists proved to be successful and would lead widespread discrimination towards Asians. Countries around the world would institute immigration laws specifically targeting Asians, particularly Chinese and Japanese persons. These laws would serve to keep Asians from immigrating to Western countries such as the U.S. Immigration Act of 1917 and The Immigration Act of 1924, among others.

Eugenics in Science & Medicine

It would be in the fields of science and western medicine that Eugenicists would make the most headway. Through genetic research, (often backed by government and private corporate funding), Eugenicists would search for scientific validation of their white supremacy. The Cold Spring Harbor Laboratory would serve as the hub for Eugenicists from all around the world to document and explore heredity within families and between races just as Galton instructed.

Cold Spring Harbor Laboratory was founded in New York in 1890. In 1904, the same year of Galton's infamous speech at the Sociological Society, Charles Davenport, the director of the Biological Laboratory at CSH, would use his position and influence to convince the Carnegie Institution of Washington (CIW) to fund the Station for Experimental Evolution (SEE) at CSH. The Carnegie Institution of Washington (CIW) would eventually fund the endeavor and Davenport became the director of the SEE. Davenport was very dedicated to promoting Eugenics and worked hard to establish it as a science. Alongside his work at CSH he also acted as Director of the American Breeder's Associations' Eugenics Committee.

In 1910, the CIW would establish Eugenics Record Office (ERO), again, under the encouragement of Davenport. This time Davenport was able to secure a grant from Marry Harriman, the widow of Edward Henry Harriman, a railroad tycoon. He would also get additional funding from The Rockefeller Foundation and John H. Kellogg and other private eugenics supporters (private "philanthropists" have always been highly involved in the promotion of the Eugenics movement). In 1921, the SEE and ERO were combined into the CIW Department of Genetics and Davenport would act as

Director until his retirement in 1934, thirteen years later (14).

Davenports' Assistant, Harry H. Laughlin, was also a pioneering member of the modern Eugenics cult. Respected for his knowledge and commitment to the Eugenics movement, Laughlin was appointed as an "expert eugenics agent" to the U.S. Congress Committee on Immigration and Naturalization. It was through his involvement in Congress that he was able to influence the passing of the Immigration Act of 1924.

A staunch supporter of compulsory sterilization in the U.S., Laughlin would write a proposal in 1922 entitled; "Eugenical Sterilization in the United States", to promote the sterilization of those deemed feeble-minded, insane, and criminal. He also promoted sterilization for epileptics, alcoholics, the deaf, deformed, and indigenous persons. As a result of his efforts, over 20 U.S. states would pass mandatory sterilization laws based upon Laughlin's suggestions. Laughlin's positions on sterilization appealed to Nazi leaders in Germany and his proposal would serve as a basis for the passing of the "Law for the Prevention of Hereditary Diseased Offspring" in 1933. Over 300,000 persons were sterilized in Germany under this law (15). In 1936, Harry Laughlin was awarded an honorary Doctorate of Medicine degree from the University of Heidelberg in Germany due to his work in "ethnic cleansing" (16).

During Davenport and Laughlin's tenure at the SEE, ERO, and the CIW Department of Genetics they would train roughly 250 field workers. These field workers, who were mainly women, had the task of gathering information from individuals regarding hereditary characteristics including physical, mental, emotional, and moral traits. This information was then logged into a "Trait Book" maintained by Davenport. Additionally, the field workers had the task of recording family traits which were also logged into record. It must be noted that much of this "data" was used by Davenport and Laughlin along with other prominent Eugenicists at the time to support legislation regarding immigration and sterilization laws around the world (14).

After facing intense scrutiny, the Eugenics Record Office (ERO) closed in 1939. The many the field workers trained there would go on and take on jobs in U.S. hospitals and mental institutions, taking their racist eugenic ideologies with them. It is no wonder that Black, Native Indian American, and Alaska Native (AI/AN) women are two to three times more likely than white women to die from pregnancy related causes in U.S. hospitals (17). Additionally, mental health care disparities in the U.S. affect mainly blacks as they often have limited access to mental health services and those available are usually of poor quality (18).

Eugenicists Strategies & Ideologies and the Effects on Societies

The U.S. Eugenics movement has gone down in history as an outdated practice ending in the late 1930's. Many people believe that the practice of Eugenics was shunned after it was used by the Nazis to justify Jewish genocide in Germany but this is far from true. These cultists just learned how to hide by looking like "peacemakers" and "philanthropists".

This is true in the case of the Jewish Holocaust. America would rush to the aid of the victims of the Holocaust making themselves appear as sympathizers. All the while, it was their eugenics ideologies that acted as the catalyst for these events. A dynamic portrait depicting "divide and conquer", a political technique that has been used in Western politics for centuries.

Similar portraits using oil-based paints, depict this strategy being used in the Middle East, namely during "Operation Cyclone" which ran from 1979-1989 (19). It was during this attempt at divide and conquer, that the United States Central Intelligence Agency (CIA), would fund rebel groups in Afghanistan. Happy to destroy their Islamic State, kill leaders, and make ruins of their infrastructure, the U.S. supplied weapons and other resources to help the rebels fight against their own Muslim brothers. It is unfortunate that many of these groups followed America in this evil affair despite having the book of Allah as a guide. Allah, The Most High, says in The Qur'an;

يَٰٓأَيُّهَا ٱلَّذِينَ ءَامَنُوٓا۟ أَطِيعُوا۟ ٱللَّهَ وَأَطِيعُوا۟ ٱلرَّسُولَ وَأُو۟لِى ٱلْأَمْرِ مِنكُمْ ۖ فَإِن تَنَٰزَعْتُمْ فِى
شَىْءٍ فَرُدُّوهُ إِلَى ٱللَّهِ وَٱلرَّسُولِ إِن كُنتُمْ تُؤْمِنُونَ بِٱللَّهِ وَٱلْيَوْمِ ٱلْءَاخِرِ ۚ ذَٰلِكَ خَيْرٌ وَأَحْسَنُ
تَأْوِيلًا

"O you who have believed, obey Allah and obey the Messenger and those in authority among you. And if you disagree over anything, refer it to Allah and the Messenger, if you should believe in Allah and the Last Day. That is the best [way] and best in result."

Surah An-Nisa, 4:59

Further,

Hazarat Abu Hurairah رَحِمَهُ ٱللَّه relates that the Holy Prophet ﷺ said:

"You are bound to hear and obey the orders of the authority, in hardship and in ease; willingly or unwillingly, and even when you are treated unjustly."

Riyad as-Salihin 667

Later, after the intended damage was done, many of those rebel groups were determined to be "terrorist" and "extremist Islamic groups" and were targeted by the U.S. military due to their threat to the world. These, and many other instances, show the cowardness of these deceptive evil doers from the Eugenics cult- they instigate evil and once the damage is done, they play the roles of sympathizer and hero who renders aid. In doing so, they can hide their true intent and appear to be the ones on the side of right. These events should serve as a stark reminder of why is important for the Muslim to adhere to their religion properly. For if you do not, the consequence is falling into the traps of Shaytan and his allies.

In the past, the Eugenics movement was more public and generally accepted. Today, on the other hand, the Eugenics cult leaders are less public and strategize in the shadows. Their public interference in the political, scientific, medical, religious, and social systems in the past has penetrated deeply in the subconscious minds and innerworkings of society both domestically and internationally. As a result, most of today's adherents to Eugenics ideologies are often less informed yet conditioned to implement the cult's strategy, often subconsciously and as a matter of "job function". This is a textbook example of the chameleon effect.

Pioneers of the Eugenics Movement & What They Left Behind

It is important to note that many of the earlier proponents of the Eugenics cult have left behind organizations that still exist today to include Margret Sangers Planned Parenthood, D.E.B Du Bois' National Association for the Advancement of Colored People (NAACP), the Rockefeller Foundation, and the Carnegie Institution among many others including the Cold Spring Harbor Laboratory. Though many mistakenly believe that the practice of Eugenics is a thing of the past, a cursory look at the research performed at the Cold Spring Harbor Laboratory even after the close of the Eugenics Record Office, would prove that to be far from the truth. Once organized, these cultists had no intention of stopping. Though the Eugenics Record Office (ERO) at Cold Spring Harbor would close in 1939, the CIW Department of Genetics under which it operated would continue its research until 1971 (20). Further, much of the earlier research done by Eugenicists at The Carnegie Institute of Washington's (CIW) Department of Genetics is being used today, as its worldwide network of cult members attempt to alter our genetic code under the guise of a "pandemic".

Continuing the Research: The Eugenics Cult & A Brief History of Their Contribution to Science & Medicine

In its 67 years of existence, the CIW Department of Genetics would play a crucial role in establishing the science of molecular genetics. The research performed there, along with other important research being done throughout the world, would set the scientific foundation for Eugenicists to implement their strategies in medicine and biotechnology. Albert Francis Blakeslee, an accomplished botanist, would succeed Davenport and become the director of the CIW Department of Genetics from 1934 to 1941. Blakeslee and his colleagues performed research on plant genetics that would make a significant impact on the study of human genetics in that it proved that certain chemicals could manipulate genes and perhaps induce mutations (21).

Milislav Demerec, a Croatian-American geneticist, became director after Blakeslee and would serve from 1941 to 1960. He would make significant contributions to the Eugenics movement through his research, which demonstrated the rudimentary ability to alter the process of natural selection through genetic interference, something Galton would have been proud of. Demerec started his P.H.D. in 1919 at Cornell University, which offered a vast variety of courses on Eugenics. His PhD work focused on maize genetics in which he was able to identify 10 different alleles that could lead to mutations in maize (22).

For reference, alleles are one of two or more versions of a particular gene which may come about via mutation. An allele that has been of particular interest to scientist is the CCR5-delta 32. This allele is a genetic mutation, which biologist believe came about as a result of plagues from the Middle Ages. The CCR5-delta 32 mutations have made 10% of Europeans resistant to HIV infection (23). Minorities, particularly African Americans, Asians, and South Americans have the lowest CCR5-delta 32 mutation rates, making them more susceptible to a wide range of diseases and viral infections, particularly HIV (24).

As I will detail later in this work, the CCR5-delta 32 allele has given Eugenics cult leaders what they believe to be "scientific proof" of their genetic superiority over other races. To Eugenicists, creating a healthier society full of what Galton described as the "best specimens" from each race, would logically involve increasing the mutation rate of the CCR5-delta 32 allele. While the mutation of the CCR5-delta 32 allele was a process of natural selection, it is my belief that COVID-19 is the Eugenics Cult attempt to create similar plague conditions like those of the Middle Ages, in conjunction with contemporary gene editing methods to increase the CCR5-delta 32 mutation rate. This increase in the mutation rate would be primarily beneficial to the white race helping them to survive and thus making them the fittest.

In 1944, bacteriologist O.T. Avery along with Colin MacLeod and Maclyn McCarty carried out experiments at the Rockefeller Institute in NY which showed that hereditary traits could be transmitted from one bacteria cell to another by *purified DNA molecules*. DNA purification via the use of a lysate is an essential first step in isolating nucleic acids, mainly DNA and RNA, from biological samples. A lysate is a mixture that will usually contain salts, detergents, and at least one nucleic acid (i.e. DNA or RNA) to act as a control. Optional ingredients might include lytic enzymes, carrier nucleic acids, and other additives. Lysates are used to isolate nucleic acids in order to prepare them for extraction (25). Avery and his colleagues described DNA as the "transforming principle", and their research would prove to be pivotal in that it brought scientists closer to understanding the mechanisms which allow genes to transmit hereditary information (26).

During Demerec's tenure as director, a scientific discovery frenzy was happening both at home and abroad. Several significant discoveries gave devoted members of the Eugenics cult hope of gaining a deeper understanding into how heredity works and further, how it might be manipulated. In order to accomplish this, scientist focused their attention to figuring out how they might reconcile Darwin's theories about natural selection with the new thoughts about heredity and population genetics. This fusion of thought would become known as *modern synthesis*. Modern synthesis was based on the ideas that 1) mutations produce various new genotypes and raw genetic materials 2) the arrangement of chromosomes affects genetic linkage 3) natural selection directs mutations.

Scientists who contributed to this new movement in scientific thought believed that humans may be able to intervene in the process of natural selection through what they called "evolutionary biology". This new type of biology would consist of understanding and manipulating 1) natural selection, 2) cell biology 3) botany 4) paleontology 5) developmental biology (i.e., embryology), 6) microbiology, 7) genomics 8) molecular biology 9) mendelian genetics 10) population genetics and 11) evolutionary ecology. In 1943, The U.S. National Research Council (NRC), formed The Committee on Common Problems of Genetics, Paleontology, and Systematics*. In one of their earlier meeting bulletins, the group discussed launching a *"synthetic attack"* on the problems of evolution (89). *(*In 1946, the committee was reorganized and became the Society for the Study of Evolution, they are still in existence today).*

These cult leaders believed that in deeply studying the disciplines mentioned above and learning how to use them to manipulate the human genome, they would be able to intervene in the process of natural selection thereby causing variations in the gene pool. The end goal would be population control through the reduction and (eventual) elimination of "problematic" races (i.e., Blacks, Native Americans, Hispanics, and other minorities) while enhancing the genetic gene pool of their own (White) race. *The study of bacteriophages would be key in unlocking those potentials. As you read through the research mentioned from this point forward, keep this important fact in mind.*

In 1941, researchers Max Delbruck and Salvador Luria met at the CIW Department of Genetics. Their work centered around bacteriophages, which are viruses that infect bacteria. Not only do these viruses infect bacteria, but they can also commandeer the machinery of the bacterial cells and multiply themselves. After hearing a lecture given by Delbruck, Demerec encouraged him to teach a series of courses on bacteriophages or "phages" for short, at the laboratory. These courses would start in 1945 and run for 26 years until 1971 (27). Phages would become a scientific specialty and ultimately Delbruck and Luria formed an international group of biologists who specialized in phages and they were often referred to as "The Phage Group" or "The American Phage Group". Phages would prove particularly relevant to the eugenicist's efforts in DNA extraction as they found that lysates (the mixture used to isolate DNA and RNA) can become highly unstable. However, to counteract instability and to stimulate the extraction process, it was found that *phage particles* can be used (25).

During his time at the CIW Department of Genetics, Demerec would work hard to make genetics a primary focus of research at the laboratory. In 1945, Demerec along with Esther M. Zimmer and Alexander Hollaender, published a research paper detailing the ability of x-ray light and UV rays to induce mutations (28). *It must be noted that Zimmer (whose last name was later changed to Lederberg) and Hollaender both worked for the U.S. Public Health Service and their research on x-ray and UV induced mutations took place alongside the Tuskegee Experiment. Additionally, In the 1950s, Demerec served on the genetics panel at the National Academies of Sciences' Committee on the Biological Effects of Atomic Radiation. As I will point out later in this work, in shaa Allah, it is no coincidence that 5G has emerged alongside COVID-19 as the negative effects of radiation on DNA have long been acknowledged by the U.S. Nuclear Regulatory Commission (29).*

In 1952, Alfred Hershey and Martha Chase, scientist at the Cold Spring Harbor Laboratory, published a research paper entitled; "Independent functions of viral protein and nucleic acid in growth of bacteriophage". Through their research, they discovered that the DNA of a virus needs to enter a bacterium in order to infect it (30). Their research would back up that of O.T. Avery and his colleges and further prove DNA was truly the transforming factor. During their research, they used radioactive sulfur and phosphorus to differentiate between viral proteins and viral DNA. They observed that radioactive phosphorus entered the bacterium increasing the replication rate of the virus giving it more control over the protein making functions of the cell.

Also known as P-32, radio phosphorus is a radioactive form of sodium phosphate. Listed below are the ingredients in the PFIZER-BIONTECH Covid-19 Vaccine:

---

mRNA, lipids ((4-hydroxybutyl)azanediyl)bis(hexane-6,1-diyl)bis(2-hexyldecanoate), 2 [(polyethylene glycol)-2000]-N,N-ditetradecylacetamide, 1,2-Distearoyl-sn-glycero-3-phosphocholine, and cholesterol), potassium chloride, monobasic potassium phosphate, sodium chloride, **dibasic sodium phosphate dihydrate**, and sucrose (31).

Notice anything familiar? Firstly, many of the ingredients listed constitute a perfect lysate mixture. Secondly, **dibasic sodium phosphate dihydrate is 32P-labeled, meaning it is a *radioactive* form of sodium phosphate** (32). Not only is this compound considered highly toxic, but it also can help COVID-19 replicate itself and take over the genetic instructions of opportunistic bacterial cells, namely NTHi. Now armed with the know-how on how to manipulate genes via bacteriophages, x-ray light, and UV rays alongside the identification of DNA as the structural chemical of interest, Eugenicists were ready for the next step in their plan to intervene in the process of natural selection, which included understanding DNAs structure.

Before joining the CIW Department of Genetics at Cold Spring Harbor Laboratory, Salvador Luria worked at Indiana University as a PhD advisor. One of his most distinguished students at the University was a Chicagoan named James D. Watson who, along with Francis Crick, would go on to discover the sequence of DNA in 1953. During his time at Indiana University, Watson was introduced to bacteriophages by Luria. He also had two other mentors who made a great impact upon his academic endeavors. One of those mentors was a geneticist named Herman J. Miller. Miller is best known for his work detailing the genetic effects of radiation. In 1926, he performed two experiments using varied doses of x-rays and was able to make a precise quantitative correlation between radiation and lethal mutations. He detailed his findings in a research paper entitled; "The Problem of Genetic Modification" (33). Miller was also a dedicated proponent of eugenics and established a biology club to promote his beliefs.

Watson's other mentor was a biologist named Tracy Sonneborn. Sonneborn devoted his career to studying the mechanisms of genetic inheritance which Watson would ultimately devote his pursuits to later in his career as well (34).

Luria saw Watson as a bright protégée who would contribute greatly to the study of bacteriophages. Luria believed that in order to propel the science of bacteriophages forward, sound knowledge of chemistry would be necessary, so Luria helped Watson obtain a post doctorial fellowship to study Chemistry in Copenhagen in 1950. In 1951, Watson enrolled in Cambridge University and would become a post-doctoral student in Cavendish Laboratory. There he would meet Francis Crick, whom he would ultimately share a Nobel Peace Prize within 1962 (35).

Watson would become the director of Cold Spring Harbor Laboratory in 1968 and would remain so for 26 years until 1994. Afterwards he would serve as the President from 1994-2003, and Chancellor from 2003-2007 (36). Though Watson was able to keep his Eugenics Cult membership partially concealed during the earlier part of his career, he was not able to maintain the façade in his older years.

Allah, The Most High, says in The Qur'an;

أَمْ حَسِبَ ٱلَّذِينَ فِى قُلُوبِهِم مَّرَضٌ أَن لَّن يُخْرِجَ ٱللَّهُ أَضْغَـٰنَهُمْ

وَلَوْ نَشَآءُ لَأَرَيْنَـٰكَهُمْ فَلَعَرَفْتَهُم بِسِيمَـٰهُمْ ۚ وَلَتَعْرِفَنَّهُمْ فِى لَحْنِ ٱلْقَوْلِ ۚ وَٱللَّهُ يَعْلَمُ أَعْمَـٰلَكُمْ

"Or do those in whose hearts is disease think that Allah would never expose their [feelings of] hatred? And if We willed, We could show them to you, and you would know them by their mark; but you will surely know them by the tone of [their] speech. And Allah knows your deeds."

Surah Muhammad, 47:29-30

'Uthman bin 'Affan (may Allah be pleased with him) said;

"Never would one conceal a secret, but Allah will expose it by the look on his face and the uncontrolled words of his tongue."

Tafsir Ibn Kathir

Towards the end of his career, Watson would make several "slips of the tongue" uncovering his racist views as it pertains to human genetics. In 2007, Watson told a *Sunday Times* reporter that he was *"inherently gloomy about the prospect of Africa" because "all our social policies are based on the fact that their intelligence is the same as ours – where all the testing says not really."* (37). According to its website, The Cold Spring Harbor Laboratory condemned these statements and claimed to have stripped Watson of all his duties at the laboratory (38).

The most telling would come in a PBS documentary

celebrating his scientific achievements in which he expressed his beliefs that data from IQ test reveal that whites are genetically more intelligent than blacks. Although Watson has been "outed" as a racist who used science to support his white supremacy beliefs, he still holds a Nobel Peace Prize, honorary doctorate degrees, and various other prizes and awards for his work. Despite their public decry of Watson, Cold Spring Harbor Laboratory still has him listed as Chancellor Emeritus on their website as of May 1, 2021, denoting his honorary retirement of duties.

After the discovery of the structure of DNA, more important scientific discoveries would be made. In 1955, Joe Hin Tijo, a research at the National Institutes of Health (NIH) began to examine the chromosomes of cancer cells. Chromosomes are long DNA molecules which contain part or all the genetic material of a particular organism. Tijo's theory was that chromosome abnormalities correlated to malignant growth and determining the exact number of chromosomes would be essential in the quest to prove his hypothesis. After studying the chromosomes in human embryonic lung fibroblasts, Tijo discovered that all unbroken cells contain exactly 46 chromosomes (39). This discovery was vital to Eugenicists as it would further enable them to implement their plot of altering DNA because now, certain chromosomes could be identified and targeted for gene deletion and translocation experiments.

Also in 1955, an American biochemist named Arthur Kornberg of Washington University School of Medicine in St.

Louis and his colleague Severo Ochoa of New York University, was able to isolate DNA polymerase (DNA's copying enzyme) from E. coli bacteria. Perhaps the most interesting thing about this discovery, (besides the discovery itself), was the materials used in the experiment. Kornberg and his team added the DNA polymerase to a tube of salt solution which also contained DNA molecules, and nucleotide building blocks, and **new DNA strands formed** (40).

The FDA and CDC have been forerunners in promoting the safety of mRNA COVID-19 vaccines. Each organization has posted seemingly harmless statements via their websites expressing that the COVID-19 vaccines approved for emergency use contain mainly lipids, salts, sugars, and buffers knowing full well these ingredients have the ability to synthesize new strands of DNA.

Now with the ability to isolate and identify particular chromosomes, the next critical discovery would be made. In 1956, Vernon Ingram, a German-American professor of biology at The Massachusetts Institute of Technology, would pinpoint the specific biological mechanisms which caused sickle cell anemia. He discovered that the disease came about due to a change in the structure of hemoglobin- particularly the substitution of valine for glutamic acid in the sixth amino acid in beta globin (41). This mutation is an example of Allah's system of natural selection as sickle cell anemia actually developed, mainly in African countries, to protect against malaria (42).

Eugenicists, however, did not see it this way. They saw

anemia, which is a disease that mainly affects those whose ancestors come from sub-Saharan Africa; regions in the Western Hemisphere (South America, the Caribbean, and Central America); Saudi Arabia; India; and Mediterranean countries such as Turkey, Greece, and Italy (43), as proof of these groups' genetic inferiority. More than 75% of the global burden of SCA occurs in sub-Saharan Africa and the only "curative" therapy offered is stem cell transplantation which now involves gene therapy. It has been widely established that children with sickle cell anemia have an increased risk for invasive bacterial infections, particularly from organisms like Streptococcus pneumoniae and Haemophilus influenzae type b (44). However, a person with any type of anemia, even a mild case, may be particularly at-risk with an invasive NTHi and COVID-19 co-infection due to the body's immune response.

As I mentioned in my research, when the body is alerted of a NTHI/COVID-19 co-infection it will progress to a nutritional immunity stage which sequesters iron. Iron is then re-introduced during the inflammation stage. These sharp rises and falls in iron for a person with anemia can be life threatening. *The creation of a bacteriophage targeting NTHi would naturally have severe effects on all of society but particularly those with anemia and other pre-existing conditions.*

To pinpoint the target of such an attack, one only needs to look at those who are primarily affected. According to the CDC, Blacks/African Americans, Hispanic/Latino

Americans, American Indian, Alaska Natives, and Asians;

- Constitute 1-2 times more cases of COVID-19 than White Americans;
- Are 1-4 times more likely to be hospitalized due to COVID-19 complications than White Americans;
- Are 1-2 times more likely to die from COVID-19 complications than White Americans (45).

In 1958, picking up from the research performed by Kornberg and his colleagues, researchers Matthew Meselson and Franklin Stahl from the California Institute of Technology in Pasadena, California would discover important mechanisms involved in DNA replication in E. coli. They made three especially important discoveries:

1. The nitrogen of a DNA molecule is divided equally between two subunits which remain intact through many generations.

2. Following replication, each daughter molecule receives one parental subunit.

3. The replicative act results in molecular doubling.

Below is an illustrative depiction of their findings using the *Watson-Crick Model*.

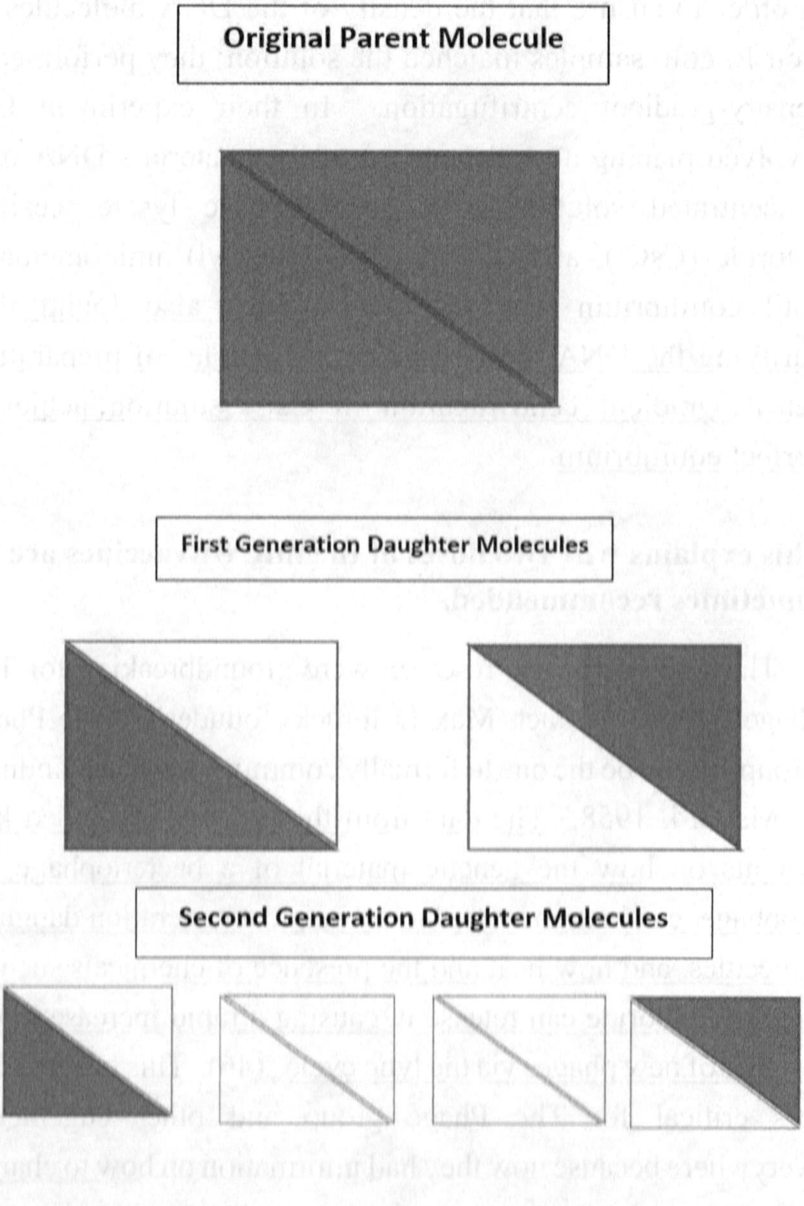

In order to reach these conclusions, the researchers employed several techniques. First, they knew that the macro molecules of DNA would be driven to the region where the solution density would be equal to their own buoyant density. In order to ensure that the density of the DNA molecules in their E. coli. samples matched the solution; they performed a density-gradient centrifugation. In their experiment this involved placing a small amount of the bacteria's DNA in a concentrated solution of dodecyl sulfate lysate, cesium chloride (CsCl), and M tris(hydroxymethyl) aminomethane until equilibrium was achieved. They also found that purifying the DNA by performing two cycles of preparative density-gradient centrifugation in CsCl solution. achieved perfect equilibrium.

This explains why two doses of the mRNA vaccines are sometimes recommended.

The findings in this research were groundbreaking for The Phage Group. In fact, Max Delbruck, founder of The Phage Group, would be the one to formally communicate these findings on May 14, 1958. The data from this research provided key insights on how the genetic material of a bacteriophage, or prophage, can be transmitted to subsequent generation daughter molecules, and how heat and the presence of chemicals such as salts and chloride can release it, causing a rapid increase in the number of new phages via the lytic cycle. (46). This information was critical for The Phage group and other eugenicists everywhere because now they had information on how to change and organism's genome through bacteriophages using the hosts own opportunistic bacteria.

The problem, however, is that not all bacteriophages cause lysogeny (i.e., virulent phage), meaning these viruses do not integrate within the host bacterium's genome. There are phages that do integrate their genomes into their host bacterium's chromosome, and these are called *temperate phages*. Though temperate phages can integrate their genome into the genome of their host, they rarely are able to cause lysis (the disintegration of a cell by rupture of the cell wall or membrane). In this way, temperate bacteriophages can integrate its nucleic acid into the host bacterium's genome or form a circular replica in the bacterial cytoplasm while the bacterial cells can continue to live and function normally (47).

Temperate phages work particularly well with Gram-negative bacteria like NTHi for exactly that reason. The cell wall of a Gram-negative bacterium is thinner than that of a Gram-positive bacterium which makes penetration of its cell wall much easier. It is well established that some methods of controlling the function of bacteria depends on the properties of the cell wall. The cell wall of Gram-negative bacteria consists mainly of Lipopolysaccharides (LPS), an endotoxin which is released when the cell wall of dead bacteria is broken down. LPS consists of polysaccharides and lipid A. Lipid A is responsible for the toxic properties that make any invasive Gram-negative infection a potentially serious medical emergency. To circumvent this, COVID-19 vaccines might act as a mechanism to deliver lipids to the bacterium in order to keep NTHi from completely dying so that it can continue function normally and continue to produce genetic material. This would allow COVID-19's genetic material to replicate within NTHi's genome giving it the ability to 1) control gene expression by stimulating the lytic cycle; 2) control transcription; and 3) control the translation process. The lipid content of COVID-19 vaccines might also serve as part of the density-gradient centrifugation allowing rapid sediment of mRNA as the Gram-negative bacteria has an asymmetric arrangement of phospholipids (48).

However, if the cell wall of Gram-negative bacteria were to become digested away, it would become a spheroplast, which have both a cell membrane and most of the outer membrane. It has been found that mRNA transcription levels are increased after the conversion of a bacterium's cell wall to a spheroplast (49). In this scenario, and the one previously mentioned, the host's genome would undergo alteration.

Taking these facts into consideration, it becomes clear why NTHi was chosen for this gene editing experiment:

1. COVID-19 (a temperate bacteriophage) will not completely destroy the cell wall of NTHi. This allows NTHi to continue functioning as NTHi and COVID-19 join to become a lysogen, allowing COVID-19 to replicate, as COVID-19 becomes a prophage.
2. mRNA COVID-19 vaccines are able to disguise prophage inducing chemicals as seemingly harmless ingredients (i.e. salts, chloride, lipids).

Additionally, it has been found that genes encoding high molecular weight adhesion proteins of NTHi are part of important gene clusters, specifically Hmw1 and hmw2 genes which encode B ORFs and C ORFs of NTHi (50). A study bacteriophage HP2 of Hemophilus influenza has demonstrated the ability of prophages to inhibit gene expression (51). These factors make NTHi an easy and viable target for a covert gene editing experiment.

For brevity, I will summarize other major discoveries since 1958 that would help Eugenicists move their "synthetic attack" plots forward into the 21st century.

- 1959: Chromosome Abnormalities (Down Syndrome, Turner's Syndrome, Intersexuality) Identified (52-54).
- 1960-1962: Berwind Peterson Kaufmann became director of the Carnegie Institution of Washington (CIW) Department of Genetics.
- 1961: Researchers Sydney Brenner, Francois Jacob, and Matthew Meselson* discovered that mRNA is the molecule that puts DNA instructions into action. *Meselson was also the researcher involved in discovering the DNA replication mechanisms in E. coli in 1958.*
- 1961: First Metabolic Defect Test for Newborns Given. Newborns tested for excess phenylketonuria (PKU) due to its ability to cause mental retardation (55).
- 1962-1971 Alfred Day Hershey became director of the Carnegie Institution of Washington (CIW)

Department of Genetics.

- 1966: Genetic Code Discovery: Over the course of several years, Marshall Nirenberg, Har Khorana and Severo Ochoa and their colleagues cracked the genetic code.
- 1968 James D. Watson became director of The Cold Spring Harbor Laboratory.
- 1968: First Description of Restriction Enzymes. Restriction enzymes are found in bacteria and have the ability to recognize and cut specific sequences of DNA (56-57). *What is quite interesting is that restriction enzymes from Hemophilus influenzae and purification methods contributed to this research.* It was found that denatured DNA along with the introduction of native phage T7 DNA as a substrate was able to produce viable DNA strands with inactive restriction enzymes (58). Once again, members of The Phage Group at Cold Spring Harbor Laboratory were involved in these discoveries including Salvador Luria.
- 1970: The Carnegie Institution of Washington's (CIW) Department of Genetics loses its name and is now generally referred to as Cold Spring Harbor Laboratory.
- 1972: First Recombinant DNA Molecules Produced using Restriction Enzymes. Recombinant DNA technology involves fusing the DNA of several species together and inserting that combination DNA into a host cell, usually a bacterium. Paul Berg, a

biochemist at Stanford who was involved in this discovery was so worried about the long-term implications that he, along with other researchers, wrote to the National Institutes of Health (NIH) asking them to regulate the use of recombinant DNA technology. They also urged other researchers to stop using the technology until it could be deemed safe. The NIH would eventually respond by creating a set of guidelines entitled; "Guidelines for Research Involving Recombinant DNA Molecules" (59-61).

- 1973: Cloning of the first animal gene (62).
- 1975-1977: Rapid DNA sequencing methods for bacteriophages discovered (63-65).
- 1976: Genentech- the First Genetic Engineering Company Founded. Genentech was founded by Herbert Boyer, one of the persons involved with the discovery of recombinant DNA technology, and a businessman named Robert Swanson. In 1977, Genentech discovered how to use bacteria to make human proteins for the treatment of diabetes. In this process DNA might be obtained from an insulin producing cell (i.e. a pancreatic cell). The insulin gene would then be isolated and injected into a bacterial plasmid. The plasmid containing the human gene would then be introduced into a bacterium which would begin to produce the insulin protein. This company would eventually expand to include about 9000 companies.
- 1977: The Discovery of Introns. Researchers

discovered that some genes in certain cells have introns which are "interruptions" or non-coding regions of the RNA transcript or the DNA encoding it. They also found that these introns are eliminated before translation through interference with the cell's mRNA (66-69).

- 1981-1982: First Transgenic Animals. Mice and fruit flies would be the first animal/insect used in the development of genetic modification methods. This is partly because mice and human genomes are remarkably similar. One of the methods to create transgenic mice includes injecting a transgene into the mouses genome during fertilization. During fertilization pre-existing mRNAs supplied by the mother are absorbed by ribosomes, new proteins are then quickly produced. There is a small window of time after the sperm reaches the egg that the maternal and paternal DNA are separated. During this time, the set of DNAs are called "pronuclei". Researchers discovered that by injecting many copies of the transgene directly into the fathers pronucleus, the transgene was integrated into embryo's chromosome. Fruit flies were particularly interesting because they could be used to study and create ways to reduce the prevalence of disease carrying insects and mosquito-borne diseases such as malaria. Interestingly, in 2000, scientists discovered a way to infect fruit flies with malaria giving them the ability to infect chickens with the deadly disease (70-73).

- 1982: GenBank Database Created. The world now had a global database whereby scientists can share DNA sequences from a variety of organisms.
- 1985: The Human Genome Project is proposed by the U.S. Department of Energy (DOE), National Institutes of Health (NIH), and other international groups including Cold Spring Harbor Laboratory. The goal: map and sequence the human genome.
- 1987: YACs Developed. Yeast artificial chromosomes (YAC) are human engineered DNA molecules used to clone DNA sequences in yeast cells. These cells are then injected into bacterial plasmid and is often used in the mapping and sequencing of genes. The use of YACs makes cloning large sequences of DNA easier (74).
- 1988: The NIH Establishes the Office of Human Genome Research. Elke Jordon is appointed Director and James D. Watson is appointed Associate Director.
- 1990: The Human Genome Project Begins. James D. Watson is appointed as Director. He was later succeeded by Francis Collins, who became the director of the NIH in 2009 and remains so today. The DOE and NIH published a plan for the first five years of the project which included:
  - Mapping & sequencing the human genome
  - Mapping & sequencing the genomes of certain organisms
  - Collect & distribute genetic data

- Study the ethical, legal, and social implications of genetic research
- Develop innovative technologies
- Transfer those technologies to the private sector for production (75)

- 1990: Research on Bacterial Artificial Chromosomes (BACs) Begins. BACs genetically engineered molecules used to clone DNA sequences in bacterial cells. These molecules are used by geneticists to study positive strand RNA viruses like COVID-19 (76).
- 1991: Expressed-Sequencing Tags (ESTs) used to Identify Gene Transcripts. ESTs is a portion of DNA sequence that is created by replicating a piece of an mRNA molecule (77).
- 1994-2003: Bruce Stillman becomes the Director of Cold Spring Harbor Laboratory. He became CEO in 2003 and remains in that position today.
- 1994: Human Genetic Map Completed. The Human Genome Project completed a detailed genetic map which allowed the scientific community to identify the specific location of certain genes (78).
- 1994: The Department of Energy (DOE) launches the Microbial Genome Project. *The goal of this project was to sequence the genomes of bacteria.*
- 1995: Haemophilus influenzae and Mycoplasma genitalium Genomes Sequenced by The Institute for Genomic Research (79-80).
- 1996: International Strategy Meeting. This was the

first international meeting to develop a strategy on human genome sequencing. Scientists from Europe, North America, and Asia discussed future projects and funding. They also agreed to make their research data available to the public.

- 1996: Mouse Genome Map Completed. This was an important milestone in helping geneticists better understand the physical origins of disease in the human genome (81).
- 1996: Yeast Genome Sequenced.
- 1996: Expressed Sequence Tags (ESTs) allow researchers to identify gene expression in a specific cell (82).
- 1996: Human Gene Map Created which displays over 16,000 locations of ESTs (83).
- 1997: The Task Force on Genetic Testing created by the NIH-DOE Working Group recommends the development of "effective" genetic testing (84).
- 2000: Yeast Two-Hybrid System Published. This system allows scientist to study protein-protein interactions in cells. It consists of altering transcription factors- which are proteins that bind to genes and turn on transcription (85).
- 2001: RNA Interference Shuts Off Mammalian Genes. Scientists found that when a cell is invaded by a double stranded RNA virus, it is recognized and cut into small pieces of RNA. These snippet RNA molecules form structures with proteins which can target similar mRNA molecules and split

them, thereby silencing the targeted gene. This experiment proved that RNA molecules could be injected into human cells and used to silence specific genes (86).

- 2001: FDA Approves Enzyme Blocking Genetics Based Drug for Leukemia (87).
- 2002: Mouse Genome Sequenced (88).
- 2003: Human Genome Project Completed.

The Human Genome Project ended in 2003 and scientists all over the world now have complete access to the human genome sequence, sequences for specific chromosomes (21 and 22), and methods for silencing and activating genes using bacteria and viruses. Though ethics committees were established along the way, this would not stop Eugenicists from using this data in the ways they deemed were appropriate for society.

A Lesson in Striving

One may ask 'why Allah, The All-Knowing, would allow such discoveries to be made considering the evil intent of these people?' The answer is quite simple as Allah says in The Qur'an;

وَأَن لَّيْسَ لِلْإِنسَـٰنِ إِلَّا مَا سَعَىٰ

"And that man can have nothing but what he strives for (good or bad)."

Surah An-Najm, 53:39

The simple fact is, these evil doers set their intentions, planned, and were diligent in their efforts. They were able to carry their plans out under the guise of government, medicine, and often with the use of taxpayer's funds. In the U.S., they polluted minority communities with poor foods, or cut off their access to healthy foods (i.e., food deserts) to promote sickness. They introduced drugs and alcohol to minorities to keep them inebriated, incarcerated, and unaware.

Through their wicked media (news, television shows, music) they controlled public perception and created illusions to keep people under a cover of darkness. While many were caught up in entertainment and pleasures (singing, dancing, chasing after the "American dream", crime, intoxicants, sexual deviance, etc.) the Eugenics Cult was left free to do their evil in plain sight!

It is most unfortunate that many Muslims have also fallen into these traps despite our having the prescriptions for righteous conduct, goodwill towards all of mankind, and the remedies for mankind's spiritual, mental, emotional, and physical disease with us (i.e., The Qur'an & Sunnah).

Muslims were once the leaders in all disciplines, particularly medicine. It is unfortunate that we have neglected this noble practice of Islamic Medicine and instead, relied upon Western Medicine. In doing so, we have placed one of our most valuable assets, our health, into the hands of Shaytan and his allies- the Eugenics Cult.

Imam As-Shafi'iy رَحِمَهُ ٱللَّه made several remarks about the noble profession of medicine. In one narration he is quoted as saying;

"Knowledge is only one of two things: Knowledge of religion and that of this world. Religious knowledge is Fiqh - Islamic Jurisprudence - while worldly knowledge is medicine."

He also said;

"I don't know anything - apart from Halal and Haraam - more noble than medicine, but, unfortunately, the people of the book have superseded us in it."

In a third narration, he expressed his disappointment towards the Muslims for neglecting the field of medicine when he said;

"They have neglected a third of knowledge and left it to the 'people of the book'.

This is why, with Allah's Aid, I founded The Halal Natural Products Academy. We offer free courses in Islamic Herbal Medicine to Muslims throughout the world. All our programs are based upon the Qur'an and Sunnah. We are training the next leaders in Islamic Medicine, and teaching them to become scientific, research-driven, analytical thinkers, who produce wholistic medicines for all of mankind, in shaa Allah.

May Allah, The Most High, forgive us and guide us back to the implementation of natural medicines according to the Qur'an and Sunnah. Ameen.

Chapter Five

DIVINE KNOWLEDGE IN THE HANDS OF THE UNRIGHTEOUS: CRISPR

RNA & Its Role in Changing the Genetic Code

While the Human Genome Project inspired most scientists around the world to focus their efforts on sequencing DNA, there was a small research group at Harvard University that wanted to explore its cousin, RNA. The group, led by biologist Jack Szostack, was piggybacking off previous research conducted in the 1980's by Thomas Cech and Sidney Altman. They would ultimately discover that some RNA could split itself and cause chemical reactions (1).

Szostack and his research team began their work by attempting to "recreate" RNA to see exactly how it can replicate itself within cells. One of the researchers on Stozstacks team was a graduate student named Jennifer Doudna. Prior to joining Stozstacks team, she had spent her academic career making DNA clones from bacteria and inserting her clones into the DNA in yeast. Together Stozstack and Doudna engineered a ribozyme that was able to make a copy of itself (2). Clearly, Doudna brought an important skillset to the table which would be important to the Eugenics Cult's mission, and she began to get noticed for it throughout the scientific community. In 1987, she was invited by James Watson to give a lecture at the Cold Spring Harbor Laboratory. Watson, someone Doudna had admired since her youth, would become her mentor throughout her career.

Doudna completed her PhD at Harvard in 1989 and has since made significant RNA discoveries *(many of these discoveries were made through studying coronaviruses)* including:

- Discovering the structure of viral RNA (3)
- Discovery of Internal Ribosome Entry Sites (IRES), which is a segment of viral RNA which can capture the ribosomes of bacterial cells and hijack them to make viral proteins (4)
- Discovery of RNA-guided gene silencing systems in bacterial cells (5)

After years of research on RNA and viral RNA, Doudna would create a technology which would enable Eugenicists finally launch their synthetic attack on mankind: CRISPR-Cas9.

CRISPR-Cas9 Discovery

Jennifer Doudna and her colleague, a French scientist named Emmanuelle Charpentier, created CRISPR-Cas9 in 2012. CRISPR-Cas9 is a technology that is used for gene editing. It allows scientists to make changes in the DNA sequences of organisms with precise accuracy. When performing research on how bacteria fight viral infections, the researchers discovered that many bacteria, like NTHi, have an adaptive immune system called CRISPR. CRISPR allows the bacteria to detect and destroy viral DNA. Within the CRISPR system there is a protein called Cas9 which can find, cut, and breakdown viral DNA in a way that can be modified. The researchers set out to better understand exactly how Cas-9 worked and in doing so, they realized that they could exploit its activity and turn it into a tool for genetic engineering (6). This technology has allowed scientists to make genetic deletions or insertions in mice, monkeys, and human embryo cells. In fact, in 2018 a Chinese scientist reported using the CRISPR-Cas9 system to silence CCR5 on human embryo cells. These children are thought to be the first "CRISPR" babies to be born (7).

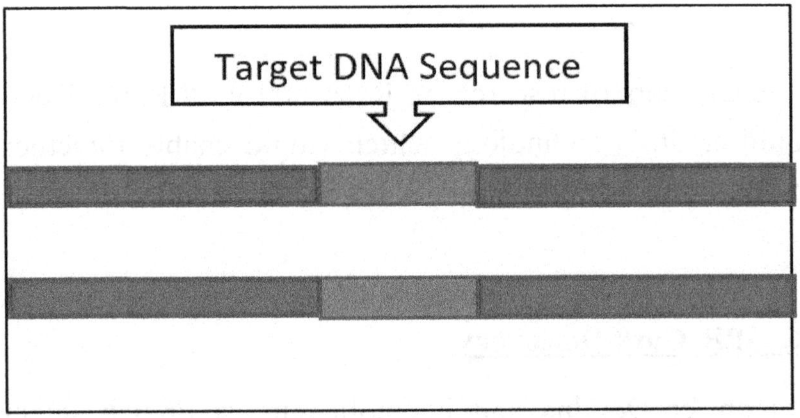

Here the guide RNA (gRNA) attaches
to the target DNA sequence.

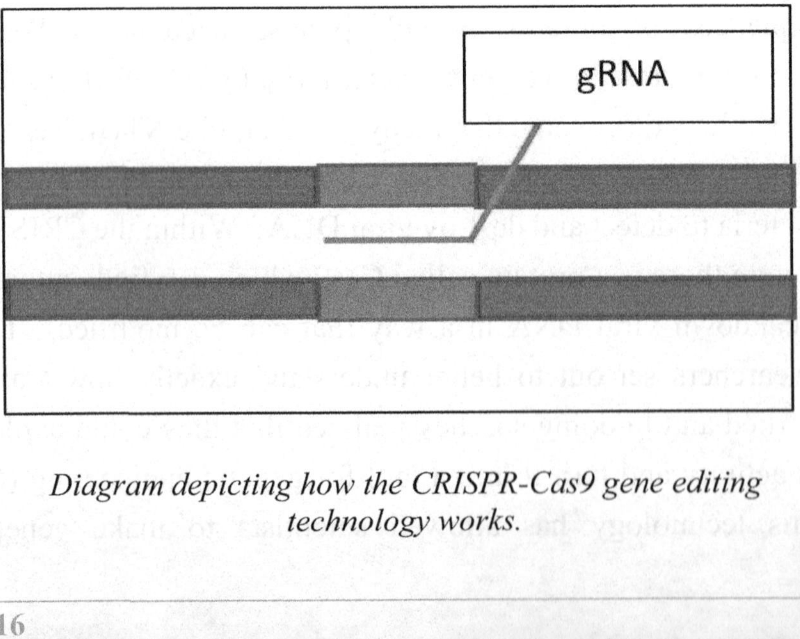

Diagram depicting how the CRISPR-Cas9 gene editing technology works.

Now the Cas9 enzyme binds to guide RNA

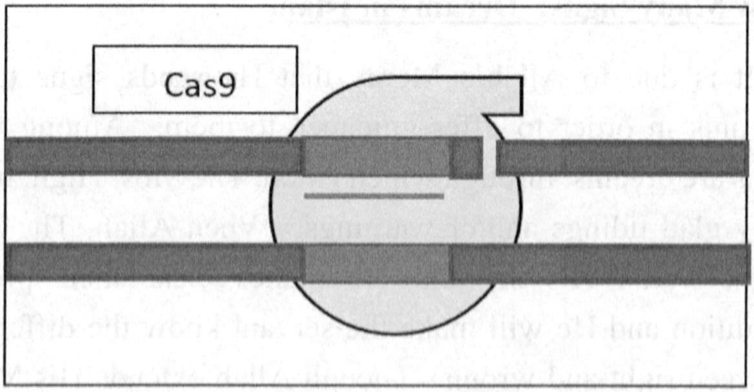

Cas9 enzyme cuts both strands of DNA

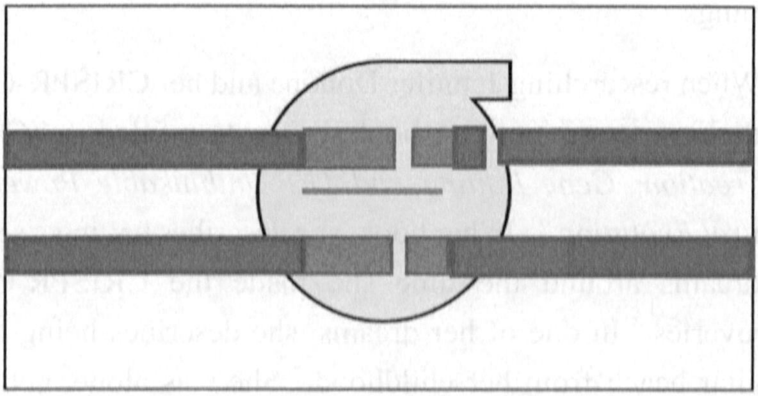

Through the DNA repair process, the cut is repaired introducing mutation.

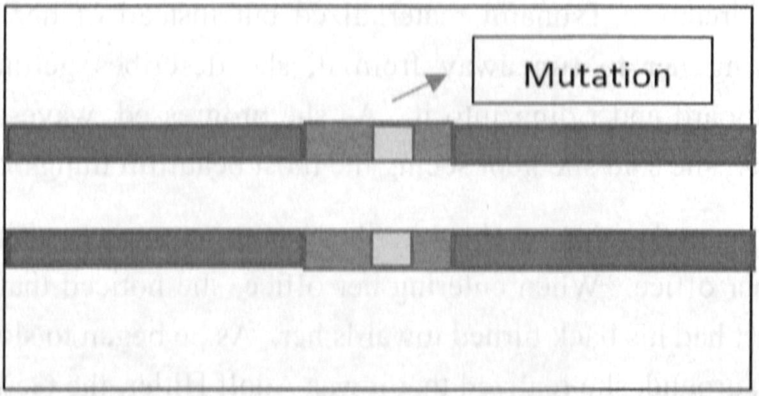

How Many Signs: Dreams in Islam

It is due to Allah's Mercy that He sends signs to his servants in order to offer guidance to them. Among these signs are dreams, through which Allah, The Most High, might relay glad tidings and/or warnings. When Allah, The Most High, warns His servant, He makes clear their present condition and He will make the servant know the difference between right and wrong. Though Allah extends His Mercy in this way, not all will take heed to His signs despite many warnings.

When researching Jennifer Doudna and her CRISPR-Cas9 technology, I came across a book she wrote entitled; *"A Crack in Creation: Gene Editing and The Unthinkable Power to Control Evolution"*. In her book, she describes having a series of dreams around the time she made the CRISPR-Cas9 discoveries. In one of her dreams, she describes being on a familiar beach from her childhood. She was alone, and the scene was picturesque. She states she was overcome by the fear of a Tsunami, a common fear she had since childhood. In her dream, a Tsunami materialized but instead of her fear driving her to run away from it, she describes getting a surfboard and riding into it. As she progressed, wave after wave, she said she kept seeing the most beautiful things.

In another dream, she describes a guest coming to visit her at her office. When entering her office, she noticed that the guest had his back turned towards her. As he began to slowly turn around, she realized that it was Adolf Hitler, the German leader responsible for the Jewish Holocaust. She claims she was overcome by fear as he asked her to tell him all about her new discoveries (8). Reading about her dreams made me think of the ayah in which Allah, The Exalted, says;

وَكَأَيِّن مِّنْ ءَايَةٍ فِى ٱلسَّمَٰوَٰتِ وَٱلْأَرْضِ يَمُرُّونَ عَلَيْهَا وَهُمْ عَنْهَا مُعْرِضُونَ

"And how many a sign in the heavens and the earth they pass by, while they are adverse therefrom."

Surah Yusef 12:105

Jennifer Doudna's dreams were most surely warnings from Allah, The Most High. The dream where she rode the waves, represented her persistence to defy natural laws by plunging into a disastrous calamity. Her curiosity fueled her determination to go further and further without inhibition, fascinated by things she saw as beautiful. Despite being in complete danger, she remained heedless and eager for more. Her meeting with Hitler is clear, this discovery would be sought after by a person or persons who have the desire to perform genocide, and they would consult with her and use her research to do exactly that.

These are the dangers of following unbelieving folk in their ways and customs. Despite their secular knowledge and seemingly high intelligence, they remain ignorant to the reality of the Lord who created them, making them unable to properly interpret His signs. How high in intelligence can one truly be if they think that the Lord of The Heavens and The

Earth and all that is in between could be man, a stone, or an animal? Despite all the knowledge that Allah has allowed them to access (i.e. the genetic code), some of them remain so ignorant that they even deny the very existence of a God!

These people are under a cover of heedlessness, they are ignorant, devoid of faith, deceptive, and their only commendable traits lie in them being methodical and persistent.

This is the danger of divine knowledge being placed in the hands of unbelievers like Jennifer Doudna. Due to their evil intentions and their desire for control and worldly possessions, their ears and hearts are mute to the signs of Allah.

We as an Ummah need to collectively organize by bringing together our own scientists, researchers, and medicine-makers who act solely according to the Qur'an and Sunnah. We are the people who are best suited to be entrusted with the affairs of science and medicine when we practice Islam properly. For when we implement Islam properly, our souls are receptive to the signs of Allah, The Most High, and closed to racism and evil intent.

Allah, The Most High, says in The Qur'an:

وَلَا تَزِرُ وَازِرَةٌ وِزْرَ أُخْرَىٰ ۚ وَإِن تَدْعُ مُثْقَلَةٌ إِلَىٰ حِمْلِهَا لَا يُحْمَلْ مِنْهُ شَيْءٌ وَلَوْ
كَانَ ذَا قُرْبَىٰ ۗ إِنَّمَا تُنذِرُ الَّذِينَ يَخْشَوْنَ رَبَّهُم بِالْغَيْبِ وَأَقَامُوا الصَّلَاةَ ۚ وَمَن تَزَكَّىٰ
فَإِنَّمَا يَتَزَكَّىٰ لِنَفْسِهِ ۚ وَإِلَى اللَّهِ الْمَصِيرُ

"And no bearer of burdens shall bear another's burden, and if one heavily laden calls another to (bear) his load, nothing of it will be lifted even though he be near of kin. You (O Muhammad ﷺ) can only warn those who fear their Lord unseen, and perform As-Salat. And he who purifies himself (from all kinds of sins), then he purifies only for the benefit of this own self. And to Allah is the final Return of all.

Surah Al-Fatir, 35:18

That is because Muslims are the best people Allah has raised up for mankind as Allah, The Most High, says in The Qur'an:

كُنتُمْ خَيْرَ أُمَّةٍ أُخْرِجَتْ لِلنَّاسِ تَأْمُرُونَ بِٱلْمَعْرُوفِ وَتَنْهَوْنَ عَنِ ٱلْمُنكَرِ وَتُؤْمِنُونَ
بِٱللَّهِ ۗ وَلَوْ ءَامَنَ أَهْلُ ٱلْكِتَـٰبِ لَكَانَ خَيْرًا لَّهُم ۚ مِّنْهُمُ ٱلْمُؤْمِنُونَ وَأَكْثَرُهُمُ ٱلْفَـٰسِقُونَ

"You [true believers in Islamic Monotheism, and real followers of Prophet Muhammad ﷺ and his sunnah (legal ways, etc.)] are the best of peoples ever raised up for mankind; you enjoin Al-Ma'ruf (i.e. Islamic Monotheism and all that Islam has ordained) and forbid Al-Munkar (polytheism, disbelief, and all that Islam has forbidden), and you believe in Allah. And had the people of the Scripture (Jews and Christians) believed, it would have been better for them; among them are some who have faith, but most of them are Al-Fasiqun (disobedient to Allah – and rebellious against Allah's Command).

Surah Ali Imran, 3:110

Western Cures for Spiritual Dis-ease

In 2008, a letter was published in *Nature* discussing the global trends in emerging infectious disease (EID). Under the direction of Peter Daszak, President of the Eco. Health Alliance, the researchers analyzed a database of 335 EID events which occurred between 1940-2004. Their research showed emerging diseases mainly consisted of those that originate in wildlife and bacteria. They also noted a correlation between the rise in EID events and the HIV pandemic and attributed this to socio-economic, environmental, and ecological factors. They further noted that EIDs place a huge burden on global economics and public health and that methods need to be employed in order to control EID to prevent global economic collapse and widespread disease (9).

One such method that has since been developed to combat EIDs is the performance of "Gain of Function" experiments. In fact, these experiments were one of the main goals of the Human Genome Project. During these experiments, scientists make modifications to viruses to make them deadlier and more transmissible. This is often done to examine how the virus might enter into human cells and spread throughout the body, allowing scientists to create vaccines and other therapeutics to treat potential disease (10).

These experiments are very risky and often undergo much scrutiny before they receive approval to start. The Wuhan Institute of Virology in Wuhan, China was one of the primary locations for Gain of Function research (11-12). Daszak and his company Eco Health Alliance received grant monies from the National Institute of Health to conduct Gain of Function experiments at the Wuhan Institute of Virology and their grant was only (temporarily) stopped once COVID-19 was declared a pandemic. Due to this, many people from the scientific community believe that COVID-19 was engineered in Wuhan however, this fact cannot be proven because the research documents are sealed. What is most interesting is that Francis Collins, former member of the Human Genome Project and now the Director of the National Institutes of Health, approved of the funds for this research. Daszak has been very vocal since the start of the pandemic in declaring that COVID-19 did not escape from the lab in Wuhan (13). Further, the World Health Organization made him (Daszak) a principal inspector into the possible leak in Wuhan which is completely bias and shows the far-reaching influence this cult has (14).

It is unfortunate that the Eugenics Cult is attempting to solve spiritual problems (i.e, sexual deviance and Shirk) through genocide and changing the fundamental elements of human composition through genetic engineering.

In Muslim countries that abide by the Qur'an and Sunnah, we do not see the prevalence of these physical and spiritual problems like in the West. This is because we denounce sexual deviance and apply the proper Shariah laws when appropriate. This is because in Muslim countries, Gods law, is law. Thus, the STD and crime rates are close to non-existent compared to Western societies. These are some of the blessings of Islam.

It is also unfortunate that many of our Muslim leaders have trusted these evil doers in the matter of COVID-19 vaccines. Prophet Muhammad ﷺ surely spoke the truth when He said;

"You would tread the same path as was trodden by those

before you inch by inch and step by step so much so that if they had entered into the hole of the lizard, you would follow them in this also. We said: Allah's Messenger, do you mean Jews and Christians (by your words) "those before you"? He said: Who else (than those two religious groups)?"

Sahih Muslim Book 47, Hadith 7

May Allah, The Most High, forgive the believing men and women. Ameen.

Chapter Six

COVID-19: CRISPR-CAS9 IN VIVO

It is my belief that COVID-19 is an attempt to intervene in the process of natural selection through the simulation of plague-like conditions from the Middle Ages in order to trigger a CCR5 delta-32 mutation via a CRISPR-Cas9 gene editing system. The CCR5 delta-32 mutation makes its carriers resistant to diseases like HIV, Smallpox, The Bubonic Plague (Black Death) (1), and most likely COVID-19. As previously mentioned, the CCR5 delta-32 mutation is more prevalent in the Caucasian population as 1% of them have two copies of the mutation and up to 20% of them have at least one copy of the mutation. In the U.S., Canada and Australia, the frequency amongst Caucasians is 8% to 10%, but less than 1% in African American populations (2). Consequently, COVID-19 is particularly harmful to African Americans and other minority groups due to the low prevalence of the CCR5 delta-32 mutation and pre-existing conditions like anemia, diabetes, heart dis-ease, and cancer. There are many CRISPR-Cas9 CCR5 editing systems that exist, however there is one which was created by scientists at Harvard University that would (in my opinion) offer the most comprehensive and effective tools to carry out a large-scale experiment like COVID-19.

Harvard's CCR5 delta-32 Patent* ***(*Funded by the NIH)***

On August 18, 2020, Harvard University was granted a patent for its CCR5 gene editing systems, by the United States Patent and Trademark Office. Their systems involve several methods and chemical compositions which can cause "loss-of-function" to CCR5. One of these systems suggest use of the CRISPR-Cas9 gene editing tool to cause a loss-of-function to CCR5 via mutation. According to the researchers, this may be accomplished by introducing the CRISPR-Cas9 system via mRNA virus particles. Further, in order to promote effective gene targeting, they also suggest combining bacteriophage Mu along with a mRNA fusion (3). Unsurprisingly, evolutionary genes to proteins in bacteriophage Mu are present in the bacterial genomes of Haemophilus influenzae. Bacteriophage Mu also plays a critical role in the DNA repair process.

DNA Repair via HDR

The CRISPR-Cas9 system often uses Homology Directed Repair (HDR) to make precise edits in the genome. HDR is a system within cells that allows it to recognize and repair double stranded DNA breaks. In order to utilize this system for gene editing, a product including gRNA, Cas9, and a DNA template for up and downstream genes must be introduced to the host. This way, the cell has exact instructions on how to repair the break. Keep in mind, these instructions may include add-ons or deletions of specific genes. Now, HDR is not always guaranteed and in fact, the efficiency rate is low, as less than 10% of alleles get modified using this method. To counteract low HDR, *fusions* may be added to the product which includes cytosine base editors (CBEs) and adenine base editors (ABEs). These base editors are essential in making very small yet, precise edits within the genome. If a scientist wanted to further ensure the purity and effectiveness of HDR, they might consider adding additional fusions to the product which would increase the product purity such as the DNA glycosylase inhibitor (UGI) or the *bacteriophage Mu- derived Gam protein (Mu-GAM)* (3).

In my research paper; "COVID-19: The Plague that Strikes Behind the Ear", I identified the Mu-GAM, though I did not realize it at the time. In my paper, I described how a NTHi / COVID-19 co-infection would cause ICAM-1 to become upregulated. ICAM-1 then coordinates bonding between LFA-1 and CD4 T-Cells. LFA-1 activation causes the release of "Leukotoxin" or LtxA which is a protein secreted by the oral bacterium, Aggregatibacter acinomycetemcomitans. *LtxA is the GAM protein of the bacteriophage Mu* (3). This information provides more insight into the pathophysiology of a NTHi / COVID-19 co-infection.

In this scenario, LtxA would increase the infectivity of CD4 T-cells which would grant COVID-19 more access to CCR5 co-receptors. LxtA is secreted as part of the immune response, however in this gene editing experiment, it would facilitate effective HDR through its ability to bind to the double strand breaks thereby protecting against the degradation of the DNA in the places where the edits are made. In this way, **COVID-19 can use mechanisms and secretions elicited by the host's adaptive immune system to not only facilitate easy access to the gene target(s), but it also uses these mechanisms to carry out the gene editing procedure.** This would be thought of as brilliant to a mad scientist. However, to sane people, its just evil.

Oftentimes, the alteration of a network of genes or sequences is required in order to effectively alter the targeted gene. Harvard University's patent suggests such alterations be made in "all possible PAM sequences" in the genome in order to generate CCR5 mutations making a NTHi a perfect target for this

COVID-19 experiment due to the Pam3Cys. P6, a main feature of this system, is a dual orientation peptidoglycan-associated lipoprotein (PAL) which is part of the Tol-Pal System. P6 has long been studied as a potential vaccine antigen. It is located on the outer membrane of NTHi and when triggered, it will activate the host's Toll-like receptor 2 (TLR2). The TRL2:P6 signaling axis responds to a NTHi infection by mounting an inflammatory response in which cytokine-secreting P6 specific T-cells (i.e. IFN-y ((Th1)) and IL-17 ((Th17))) are summoned giving COVID-19 access to CCR5 co-receptors. It is during this process that the Tol-Pal compounds can facilitate the penetration of bacteriophage Mu particles (from LtxA) into NTHi. During this process transcription can occur as Aggregatibacter acinomycetemcomitans contains genes encoding the Tol-Pal system – (ybgC – tolQ – tolR – tolA)(tolB-pal-ybgF). Transcription occurs from promoters located upstream of the 5' ends of genes ybgC and tolB. This DNA sequence or "PAM motif" as described within Harvard's patent, is required for Cas9-DNA interaction (3-5).

sRNA Targets

During the inflammatory response, iron is sequestered as part of the nutritional immunity phase. In NTHi, the ferric uptake regulator (Fur) acts to regulate and balance iron levels throughout the body. Fur also can positively affect gene expression via a small RNA (sRNA) intermediate called HrrF. HrrF targets genes whose byproducts are involved in molybdate uptake, deoxyribonucleotide synthesis, and amino acid biosynthesis.

Orthologs, which are evolutionary genes of HrrF only exist in members of the Pasteurellaceae Family of which NTHi and Aggregatibacter acinomycetemcomitans are both members. *It is critical to mention the unknown dangers of editing orthologs.* These are genes which have been essentially passed down from our ancestors', generation after generation, and have retained the same function throughout that evolution. Alterations of these genes can have devastating, long-lasting effects and further, it can be *fatal*. HrrF target genes include the modABC gene cluster, asnA, asnC, and nrdB. Some of these orthologs encode major iron utilization systems including hitABC, hxuABC, hfeABCD, tbpA and tbpB, hgpB, hgpC, and hgpD. Fur regulated sRNAs in Aggregatibacter acinomycetemcomitans include JA01 though JA04 (6).

As I pointed out in my research paper, people who have iron deficient blood (anemia) have a higher risk for severe disease complications from COVID-19. This is because during the nutritional immunity phase iron is sequestered, and consequently, iron levels rapidly dip to dangerous levels. Though bad for the host, this is good for the gene editing experiment because HrrF gene expression is higher when iron levels are low. This is dangerous for those with even mild iron deficiencies, and as a reminder, *Blacks have moderate to severe anemia almost 3 times more than Whites and Hispanics.*

The Role of Radiation

In gene editing, UV radiation has several applications. For one, radiation can be used to induce mutations in combination or in lieu of the lysate administration (COVID-19 vaccines). It is also helpful in silencing specific cellular targets (i.e., genes) during the DNA repair process. However, radiation has severe health risks which have been well established. To combat the toxicity of radiation RNA interference is often used.

RNA interference (RNAi) is a technology which a cell uses its own gene DNA sequences to turn it off, this process is called silencing. During RNAi, an RNA sequence is cut into to small parts by an enzyme called a "Dicer", thereby creating small interfering RNAs (siRNA). These siRNA can now bind to the small RNAs (sRNA) like the ones found in NTHI and Aggregatibacter acinomycetemcomitans, opening the way for transcription and gene silencing. RNAi is a commonly used tool, and it is quite easy to purchase customized siRNAs from a variety of manufacturers online. This technology makes it easy to pick any gene, in virtually any organism, and design a siRNA that will silence it. It is also relatively cheap and easy to produce. Viruses, coronaviruses in particular, have long been used as a delivery technology for RNAi (7).

Radiation may be administered many ways but for a global experiment such as COVID-19, a universal technology would need to be employed. During radiation therapy, specific cells are targeted using a machine that emits beams of intense energy to kill cells. I propose that **in the COVID-19 experiment, the energy beams come from 5G radiation and the machine of choice is the cell phone.** This technology would make it easy to target the NTHi bacterium as they are usually found in the ears, nose, and throat region over 80% of all humans. Holding a 5G enabled phone to the ear would be an easy means to administer radiation in this experiment. If you think my proposition is far-fetched, think again. Jennifer Doudna, along with other researchers throughout California and Germany created a technology which would allow COVID-19 testing to be performed using the camera on a cell phone and a "florescence" detector. Their research paper entitled; "Amplification-free detection of SARS-CoV-2 with CRISPR-Cas13a and mobile phone microscopy", details this technology and was published on January 21, 2021 in *Cell.*

Further, using 5G radiation to stimulate mutation, is simply a way to counteract low vaccine adherence. It is also a method to increase the precision and silencing of the CCR5 via RNAi mechanisms.

In 2016, reports began to surface from Cuba about "strange energy attacks" seemly directed at U.S. diplomats. They called these attacks "Havana Attacks" and symptoms included; ear popping, vertigo, pounding headaches, and nausea, difficulty reading, irritability, memory and sleep problems, brain injury, and sometimes accompanied a "piercing directional noise". The U.S. Central Intelligence Agency (CIA) was accused of not taking the reports seriously until these attacks began to happen against government officials near the White House in 2019 and China and Russia began to report similar incidents. The National Academy of Sciences released a report in December 2020, about these incidents calling them "directed microwave energy attacks"

(8-9). They stated that injuries sustained from these attacks using "directed pulse radio frequency" may have aggravating causes such as chemical exposures and infectious diseases. Where I am, we have experienced two such events in the past week, the last happening just 30 minutes ago. The first incident happened on Wednesday of this week as I lay down for an evening rest. I was awakened by a loud piercing sound which I had never heard before, then our lights went out. Through my window, I could see the sun shining, no rain, no thunder. I could hear two neighbors outside discussing what might have just happened. The second incident happened right around Fajr. There was a loud "boom" as if something extremely heavy had fallen to earth, and then lights went out and quickly came back on. A look outside revealed nothing, though dark, I could see that there was no storm, there had not been a car accident which could have caused such a sound. There are incidents from around the country of people experiencing things just as I have mentioned and we all should expect for these instances to become a frequent occurrence in the days ahead. I do believe that the Eugenics Cult are not only using 5G radiation in the COVID-19 experiment, but they will also use this technology as a biological weapon, and Allah, The Most High, knows best. May Allah, The All Knowing, expose and stop these devils, Ameen.

Understanding the purpose and biological mechanisms of COVID-19 is imperative in order to prescribe the proper Islamic treatments and to understand the long-term health implications of this disease. Below I have included a template for an informed consent disclosure that I believe the Eugenics

Cult should have submitted to the world before conducting their global clinical trial. I will then present an overview of the pathophysiology of COVID-19 based upon my research findings. Keep in mind that there are many systems that may be employed to facilitate a CCR5 delta-32 mutation or a multiplex genetic experiment using CRISPR-Cas9 (i.e., COVID-19) and so my research, though relevant, only provides a limited and rudimentary view of the matter.

COVID-19: Informed Consent Disclosure

1. COVID-19 is biological terrorism event perpetrated by the Eugenics Cult against all of humanity.
2. Further, it is a Gain of Function gene editing experiment whereby:
    - All test subjects (humans) are subjected to a change in the environment due to the intentional release of a genetically engineered virus (COVID-19).
    - Purpose: Gene Silencing using the CRISPR-Cas9 Technology.
    - Primary Therapeutic Target: CCR5 delta-32 allele
    - Experiment Duration: Indefinitely
    - The primary "treatments" include:
        - o Genetically engineered virus particles containing mRNA, DNA, Cas9, lysates
        - o mRNA vaccines
        - o Radiation Therapy
    - Test subjects are placed into one of (at least) four groups:

- o Vaccinated (Treatment Group)
- o Radiation Therapy (Treatment Group)
- o Unvaccinated (Control Group)
- o No Radiation Therapy (Control Group)

3. COVID-19 is also a mass genocide attempt targeting:

- Persons of African decent
- Hispanics
- Native Americans
- Asians
- Middle Eastern persons (and in that order)

4. COVID-19 is also a is a population control effort targeting the world's poorest members namely those in;

- Africa
- India
- South America

5. Risks & Side Effects include:

- Mild, moderate, to severe reactions to virus particles which may result in long-term disease manifestations, permanent disability, and death.
- Irreversible changes to your DNA and ultimately the DNA to your unborn offspring.
- Off-target editing risk which may result in unintended chromosomal changes and birth defects.

Since this is a new experiment, not enough data has been collected to accurately assess all of the possible long-term implications. However, we do believe the benefits of this experiment greatly outweigh any associated risks as 1) not everyone will die as the "fittest specimens" from each race will naturally be preserved and 2) causing a "loss-of-function" to the CCR5 co-receptor may grant immunity to HIV and other viral diseases for the current generation and those to come. Please sign below to grant your consent to receive the treatments mentioned above and any treatments that have not been listed herein as we hereby retain the right to create and administer additional treatments without disclosure.

Participant Signature: __________ Date: ___________

COVID-19: CRISPR-Cas9 In Vivo

1. COVID-19: a genetically engineered bacteriophage of Nontypeable Haemophilus Influenzae (NTHi)- carrying gRNA (small interfering RNAs or siRNAs) enters the host.

2. NTHi identifies COVID-19 and attempts to destroy it through the upregulation of ICAM-1.

3. ICAM-1 acts as a ligand to LFA-1.

4. LFA-1 becomes active on CD4 T-cells.

5. LFA-1 activation on target and infected CD4 T-cells enhance COVID-19 infectivity and transmission by promoting virus binding and cell to cell spread via the CCR5 co-receptor. COVID-19 now has access to the CCR5 target DNA sequence within the NTHi bacterium.

6. gRNA binds to the target sequence.

7. Cas9 enzyme binds to gRNA.
8. Host is exposed to treatments;
   - Vaccines
     - Sodium, sugars, phosphate, chloride bind to Cas9 causing it to activate.
     - mRNA is introduced and causes the process of translation.
     - Cas9 functions to repress expression of the CCR5 delta-32 allele.
     - Cas9 cuts DNA
     - The cut is repaired introducing CCR5 delta-32 mutation.
     - New proteins are created from the mRNA template.
   - Radiation Therapy
     - Cas9 enzyme binds to gRNA
     - Cas9 cuts DNA
     - The cut is repaired introducing CCR5 delta-32 mutation.

<u>Implications: Evolutionary Changes to the Human Genome</u>

This COVID-19 experiment is a manifestation of one of Shaytan's loftiest goals as Allah, The Exalted, has informed us of in The Qur'an;

وَلَأُضِلَّنَّهُمْ وَلَأُمَنِّيَنَّهُمْ وَلَآمُرَنَّهُمْ فَلَيُبَتِّكُنَّ آذَانَ الْأَنْعَامِ وَلَآمُرَنَّهُمْ فَلَيُغَيِّرُنَّ خَلْقَ اللَّهِ ۚ
وَمَن يَتَّخِذِ الشَّيْطَانَ وَلِيًّا مِّن دُونِ اللَّهِ فَقَدْ خَسِرَ خُسْرَانًا مُّبِينًا

"Verily, I will mislead them, and surely, I will arouse in them false desires; and certainly, I will order them to slit the ears of the cattle, **and I will order them to change the nature created by Allah.** And whoever takes Shaitan (Satan) as a Wali (protector or helper) instead of Allah, has surely suffered a manifest loss."

Surah An-Nisa, 4:119

Attempts at CCR5 delta-32 mutations using certain base editors (i.e., AID mediated mutagenesis (TAM) and CRISPR-X) can cause evolutionary changes and hold many unknowns particularly for the next generation who may experience high rates of birth defects due to unintended alterations in chromosomal arrangements. Additionally, this experiment may be the cause for increased cancer rates due to higher levels of radiation and it can spur the emergence of new diseases. Further, it is well established that bacteria have memory that is transmittable to the next generation. In NTHI, P6 contains that memory, thus targeting the TLR2:P6 signaling axis is dangerous and will cause evolutionary changes to the human genome.

At this point, it should be quite clear that COVID-19 is a coordinated attack and further, that is its perpetrated by the Eugenics Cult. They have been planning this attack since the turn of the 20th century, and because of our collective misdeeds as a society, we have all become rightful victims. It is important to identify some of the current leaders of the Eugenics Cult so that they may be further exposed and held accountable, and all success comes from Allah, The Most High.

Chapter Seven

COVID-19: DRIVING PROFITS FOR THE 1%

Imam An-Nawawi رَحِمَهُ ٱللَّه said;

"There are some doctors who have little or no fear of Allah, who want to take more than their due, or even strip their patients of all their possessions. Nay, in fact there are some of these private hospitals which were purposely set up for material purposes only, that is to rake in profits, make-it-rich-quick. They aim to strip the patient of all his possessions and if they had the chance, they would have stripped his bones from the flesh that covers it."

Though members of the Eugenics Cult come from all races and socio-economic backgrounds, the leaders can be found amongst the world's wealthiest, the 1%. It is estimated that the 1% possess 45% of the world's wealth. They are strategically embedded within various industries where they can infiltrate systems and governments to carry out their agendas. Below I will attempt to identify some of these persons, their companies, and their government counterparts. As you will see, not only has the 1% been making sure they genetically survive during COVID-19, they also have been ensuring that they thrive financially.

The Beneficiaries & Profiteers of COVID-19

Peter Danzak, The Eco. Health Alliance, The National Institutes of Health (Francis Collins & Anthony Fauci), & The World Health Organization

Danzak is the President of Eco. Health Alliance who received grants from the NIH to perform "Gain of Function" experiments in Wuhan, China. The research his company performed there should be released to an independent board of scientists and reviewed. Currently this information is sealed. The National Institutes of Health funded much of this research and has awarded the Eco. Health Alliance over $7 in grant funding since August of 2020. Despite the conflict of interest, the World Health Organization made Peter Danzak an investigator into the origins of COVID-19 in Wuhan, China.

Bill Gates & Cold Spring Harbor

In 2020, Bill and Melinda Gates purchased 242,000 acres of land, making them the largest holder of private farmland in America (1). According to a report by Coldwell Banker, America's wealthiest people have left cities and coastal towns and have relocated in suburbs, ski towns, and vacation resorts since the COVID-19 started. This report lists 132 cities and states that the wealthy have relocated to, the top four suburbs being; East Bay, California, King County, Washington, Colorado Springs, Colorado, and Fairfax, Virginia (2-3). When Galton spoke at the Sociological Society in London, he talked of the fittest race and their necessity to procreate under environmental stress. This land purchase is to facilitate the Eugenics Cult and their members in having access to fresh air, clean water, whole foods, and housing which will make their ability to procreate with "the best specimens" from their own race easy for them when the impact of COVID-19 reaches its height. Additionally, the Gates have been active in Africa since starting their non-profit foundation in 2000. Many of their initiatives in Africa revolve around HIV/AIDS, Anemia, Malaria, and vaccine research, development, and administration. The Bill & Melinda Gates Foundation has awarded many of these grants to Cold Spring Harbor Laboratory, which has been a haven for eugenics research for over a century (4).

Cold Spring Harbor Laboratory & The Pershing Square Foundation

In 2015, just three years after CRISPR-Cas9 was created, The Pershing Square Foundation awarded a $10 million dollar grant to the Cold Spring Harbor Laboratory for its biology, genetics, and education programs (5).

Presidential Administrations, The U.S. Department of Energy & The National Institutes of Health

Bill Clinton became President of the United States in 1993, three years after the start of the Human Genome Project which was spearheaded by Department of Energy (DOE) and the National Institutes of Health. Since the start of the Human Genome Project, they have encouraged the creation of innovative genetic technologies to be produced by the private sector. Bill Clinton played a great role in furthering the eugenics movement through his support of the Human Genome Project and through starting many initiatives which would pave the way for COVID-19. When the sequence of DNA was discovered, Bill Clinton was quoted as saying; *"Today we are learning the language in which God created life."* Clinton was instrumental in paving the way for COVID-19 technology, more specifically, 5G radiation. 5G requires a massive amount of energy and investors have long eyed wind energy as a potential source. There is much bureaucracy involved in the offshore wind farm process. When a state wants to develop offshore energy sites, they must seek approval through the U.S. Department of the Interior and the Bureau of Ocean Energy Management. The DOI/BOEM will then establish a task force consisting of members from the local tribal government, state government, and federal government to assess the feasibility of the project (6). Though private industry players are often the developers, their presence at this phase is not allowed and in order to influence decision making, they need inside players especially at the federal level which has (since the start of the Human Genome Project) mainly been supplied by Presidential Administrations.

During his administration, Clinton set the groundwork for offshore wind farms and the Biden administration is now attempting to move 30,000 megawatts of electricity from offshore wind farms by 2030 (7). These moves by the Biden administration seem to be fueled by the not so coincidental Colonial Pipeline cyber-attack. The Colonial Pipeline is the main pipeline for gasoline and diesel fuel supply to the U.S. East Coast (8). Not only would offshore wind farms provide more opportunities for 5G energy, but they are also hard to penetrate by cyber-attack or physical attack due to their location in the ocean. Moving 5G energy offshore would ensure that the Eugenicist Cult leaders can administer radiation without the possibility of interruption, and Allah, The Most Wise, knows best.

Mark Zuckerberg & Facebook

Mark Zuckerberg, along with Bill Gates and Warren Buffet, signed onto the Giving Pledge which is a group of millionaires and billionaires who have pledged to give away 99% of their wealth to philanthropy in their lifetime. In order to accomplish this goal, Mark Zuckerberg and his wife, Priscilla Chan, established a non-profit called Biohub in which they plan to "cure all childhood diseases" within their lifetime through research on genomics, infectious diseases, and implantable devices (9). His company, Facebook, has also been hyperactive in removing pages which contain discouraging messages about COVID-19 vaccines (10). Much like Bill Gates, Zuckerberg has been aggressively purchasing real estate throughout the United States.

Elon Musk & The city of Starbase, TX

Elon Musk, founder of Tesla and SpaceX, is in the process of establishing a resort town in Texas (11)

Harvard University & The National Institutes of Health

Patent holder of the technology most capable and most likely used for COVID-19. They received grant funding from the NIH to perform the research relating to this technology.

mRNA Vaccines (major players):

- Pfizer & BioNTech
- Moderna
- Johnson & Johnson

Note: many countries around the world are calling for a relax on patent protections so that other manufacturers can make mRNA vaccines for poor countries. The U.S. has been against this move, most likely because the specific formula for the mRNA would be released to the general public, which would reveal the truth behind these vaccines and Allah, The Most High, knows best.

Jennifer Doudna Companies

- Mammoth Biosciences – Founded in 2017. Provides CRISPR-driven genome editing tool kits as well as other CRISPR-driven products.
- Scribe Therapeutics - Founded in 2018. Development of CRISPR based genetic medicine.

Main Companies Driving 5G Technology

- Microsoft
- Google
- Verizon
- Dell
- Motorola Solutions

World Governments

World governments, particularly those in poor countries like Africa, India, and China should also be evaluated. As this book is being written, India is facing an overwhelming COVID-19 crisis with reports of 150 persons dying every hour. New Delhi, one of the hardest hit cities by COVID-19 portrays polarized views of the rich and poor. Despite new Delhi having 46% of all its countries COVID-19 cases, Prime Minister Narendra Modi continues with a $1.8 billion renovation of its government buildings.

May Allah, The Most High, fully expose all those who are responsible for COVID-19, Ameen.

AUTHOR'S REFLECTIONS

A CALL TO TAWHEED

بسمله الرحمن الرحيم

In the name of Allah, The Most Gracious, The Most Merciful

Oh, Humanity!

We are entering into precarious times as we draw near to The Day when all souls shall return to their Lord, Allah. Evil has seeped from the souls of many men and women and has gained access to their hearts, blinding them from seeing the humanity in their fellow human being. The thought of losing the things they covet – wealth, power, and authority, grips them with such fear that they are willing to do cruel, evil things to preserve them. We must understand, oh reader, that are in essence spiritual beings, having a human experience and this Dunya (world) is not our home. We are mere travelers passing by and it is only the extremely foolish who is loaned something for a time that will try to possess it forever. The evil doers of the Eugenics Cult have been tested with intelligence, wealth, and authority in the land. Instead of using these gifts from Allah, The Most High, for good, they have become deceived by them and allowed arrogance to enter their hearts. They believe that because they have been given these blessings, it is a mark of their superiority. Futher, they believe this superiority gives them the right to make decisions that will foremost benefit themselves and their offspring. These cultists have striven for soci-economic, environmental, and biological reasons to justify their decision to commit genocide, citing population growth, global warming, infectious disease, criminality, and the global burden of the poor as indications of mankind's ultimate decline. In reality, these people are Awuliyah-Ash Shaytan (friends of the devil). Their fears and greed have led them to commit atrocities against mankind for ages. Allah, The Most High, says in the Qur'an;

ٱلشَّيْطَـٰنُ يَعِدُكُمُ ٱلْفَقْرَ وَيَأْمُرُكُم بِٱلْفَحْشَآءِ ۖ وَٱللَّهُ يَعِدُكُم مَّغْفِرَةً مِّنْهُ وَفَضْلًا ۗ وَٱللَّهُ وَٰسِعٌ
عَلِيمٌ

"Shaytan (Satan) threatens you with poverty and orders you to commit Fasha' (evil deeds, illegal sexual intercourse, sins); whereas Allah promises you Forgiveness from Himself and Bounty, and Allah is All-Sufficient for His creatures' needs, All-Knower."

Surah Al-Baqarah, 2:268

Make no mistake, even though the leaders from the Eugenics Cult are primarily those with white skin, the evil they embody is not due to their race. Their propensity towards evil is completely a matter of the heart. This type of evil can rest in the chest of any man or woman who has allowed space for arrogance, jealousy, disbelief, and greed.

For there are many people within all races who have allowed Shaytan to overcome their hearts in this same way, causing them to become an enemy to their own people! No person is exempt from "spiritual heart disease", in fact, this disease is the start to all other manifestations of disease be it spiritual, physical, emotional, or mental. We were all born with individual propensities towards evil as a test and a trial from our Lord. Therefore, sins are various and its levels are many. However, only those who turn to Allah, The Healer, can experience a complete healing as Allah, says in the Qur'an;

يَـٰٓأَيُّهَا ٱلنَّاسُ قَدْ جَآءَتْكُم مَّوْعِظَةٌ مِّن رَّبِّكُمْ وَشِفَآءٌ لِّمَا فِى ٱلصُّدُورِ وَهُدًى وَرَحْمَةٌ لِّلْمُؤْمِنِينَ

"O humanity! There has come to you a good advice from your Lord (i.e. the Qur'an, enjoining all that is good and forbidding all that is evil), and a healing for that (disease of ignorance, doubt, hypocrisy, and differences) which is in your hearts, - a guidance and a mercy (explaining lawful and unlawful things) for the believers."

Surah Yunus, 10:57

As we progress into this new age, we must understand that our collective human experience was never supposed to be a war between races. Allah, The Most High, created us so that we may learn from one another and help one another. Further, it is not our gifts or possessions that signify our rank with Allah, for He gives honor to whom He pleases. Allah, The Most High, says in The Qur'an;

يَـٰٓأَيُّهَا ٱلنَّاسُ إِنَّا خَلَقْنَـٰكُم مِّن ذَكَرٍ وَأُنثَىٰ وَجَعَلْنَـٰكُمْ شُعُوبًا وَقَبَآئِلَ لِتَعَارَفُوٓا۟ ۚ إِنَّ أَكْرَمَكُمْ عِندَ ٱللَّهِ أَتْقَىٰكُمْ ۚ إِنَّ ٱللَّهَ عَلِيمٌ خَبِيرٌ

"O mankind! We have created you from a male and a female, and made you into nations and tribes, that you may know one another (not hate one another). Verily, the most honorable of you with Allah is that (believer) who has At-Taqwa [i.e. he is one of the Al-Muttaqun (the pious)]. Verily, Allah is All-Knowing, Well-Acquainted (with all things).

Surah Al-Hujurat, 49:13

Prophet Muhammad ﷺ said;

Beware! There is a piece of flesh in the body if it becomes good (reformed) the whole body becomes good but if it gets spoilt the whole body gets spoilt and that is the heart.

Sahih al-Bukhari, Book 2, Hadith 45

Race, nationality, soci-economic factors, education, have all just been tools that Shaytan has consistently used to divide us, and truly he is an enemy to us all. Indeed Allah, The Most High, has showed mankind that He raises and lower whom He wills despite race, nationality, education, wealth, etc. We have this sign in the coming of our Prophet Muhammad, ﷺ. Allah, The Most High, chose him, an Arab to be His Messenger and Prophet. He was unlettered, (could not read) and further he was not wealthy, however, Allah endowed him with beautiful character and a pure heart, and it was through him that the only holy book that has never been changed (i.e., The Qur'an) was revealed.

We must realize that our battle in this Dunya, has never been about race. Yet it has, and always will be, a battle one between good and evil, belief and disbelief, guidance and misguidance. Our current predicament exemplifies this fact, as COVID-19 has been thrust upon us all despite our skin color. The enemy, whose heart has reached a level of spiritual deadness that many of us cannot fathom, is willing to sacrifice even those who share their skin color in order to hit their intended target. Just like an archer, our collective enemy has pulled back their bow, and let loose the arrow. Hitting any spot point on the dartboard will suffice, however every skillful archer wants to hit the bullseye.

COVID-19 is an experiment in which there are several different test groups. Every experiment has its primary test group and a corresponding therapeutic goal. In order for society to have an opportunity to defend ourselves against our collective enemy, we must analyze the target group and further, understand why they are relevant. This analysis must be done wholistically, meaning we must examine the spiritual, physical, mental, and emotional aspects of this affair. As I proceed, I will identify the primary target group for this experiment. Further, I will discuss the wholistic implications which have led to their prioritization. In the following passages, I will address this group directly however, the reader should know that this message is universal and written for all of humanity.

COVID-19 & The Chosen Ones

As I have made clear earlier in the text, it is not by chance that Blacks, Hispanics, Native Americans, and Asians suffer most and have the highest mortality rate from COVID-19. It should be clear to you by now that COVID-19 is an intentional event, and these groups sit in various positions within the bullseye, Blacks being dead in the center. These groups have been targets of oppression (i.e., slavery, genocide) at different times throughout history and there is a reason for this. You are the descendants of Bani Israel (The Children of Israel), people comprising the twelve tribes. You were the people chosen for Allah's special favors and consequently, have long been the target of hatred, jealousy, and oppression from Shaytan and his allies. What is happening now to you is the same that happened when you were enslaved by the Egyptians and Allah, The Most High, sent you a blessed messenger, Prophet Musa عَلَيْهِ ٱلسَّلَامُ. Then your enemy, Shaytan, used his allies, Fir'aun (Pharoah) and his people, to enslave you, kill your children, and rape your women folk. Shaytan's attack against you has been the same throughout history, it is only his methods that have changed form. It is no coincidence that Allah, The All Wise, arranged the Qu'ran in such a way that you are addressed very early on;

يَٰبَنِىٓ إِسْرَٰٓءِيلَ ٱذْكُرُوا۟ نِعْمَتِىَ ٱلَّتِىٓ أَنْعَمْتُ عَلَيْكُمْ وَأَنِّى فَضَّلْتُكُمْ عَلَى ٱلْعَٰلَمِينَ

"O Children of Israel! Remember My Favor which I bestowed upon you and that I preferred you to the 'Alamin [mankind and jinn (of your time period, in the past)]."

Surah Al-Baqarah, 2:47

وَإِذْ نَجَّيْنَٰكُم مِّنْ ءَالِ فِرْعَوْنَ يَسُومُونَكُمْ سُوٓءَ ٱلْعَذَابِ يُذَبِّحُونَ أَبْنَآءَكُمْ وَيَسْتَحْيُونَ
نِسَآءَكُمْ ۚ وَفِى ذَٰلِكُم بَلَآءٌ مِّن رَّبِّكُمْ عَظِيمٌ

"And (remember) when We delivered you from Fir'aun's (Pharaoh) people, who were afflicting you with a horrible torment, killing your sons and sparing your women, and therein was a mighty trial from your Lord."

Surah Al-Baqarah, 2:49

وَإِذْ فَرَقْنَا بِكُمُ ٱلْبَحْرَ فَأَنجَيْنَـٰكُمْ وَأَغْرَقْنَآ ءَالَ فِرْعَوْنَ وَأَنتُمْ تَنظُرُونَ

"And (remember) when We separated the sea for you and saved you and drowned Fir'aun's (Pharoah) people while you were looking (at them, when the sea-water covered them).

Surah Al-Baqarah, 2:50

Let this serve as glad tidings, O, humanity! Just as Allah, The Exalted, aided the Children of Israel against a mighty enemy before, He most certainly has all the Power and Strength to do it again, out of His infinite Mercy for his creatures, and Allah, does not like oppression. O, Children of Israel, you were given a great victory by Allah, The Most Kind, once before but now you are back under the grasp of your enemy. How is this so!?

This is because when Allah, The Exalted, delivered you before you were not grateful for His blessings and you were unwilling to enter his religion completely. You have always loved the ways of your oppressor- his religion, his love of wealth, his government. When you were delivered once before, Allah was most Patient and Kind with you, he understood how indoctrinated in your enemies' ways you had become. He showed you many signs, starting with the parting of the sea, to demonstrate to you His Power and His Protectiveness over you. Despite all that, you certainly gave His Messenger, Prophet Musa عَلَيْهِ ٱلسَّلَامُ a hard time. Prophet Musa عَلَيْهِ ٱلسَّلَامُ enjoined monotheism, the belief in One God (Allah) upon you but you turned back, desiring to worship the calf. Allah, The Exalted says in The Qur'an;

وَإِذْ وَٰعَدْنَا مُوسَىٰٓ أَرْبَعِينَ لَيْلَةً ثُمَّ ٱتَّخَذْتُمُ ٱلْعِجْلَ مِنۢ بَعْدِهِۦ وَأَنتُمْ ظَٰلِمُونَ

"And (remember) when We appointed for Musa (Moses) forty nights, and (in his absence) you took the calf (for worship), and you were Zalimun (polytheists and wrong-doers). Then after that We forgave you so that you might be grateful."

Surah Al-Baqarah, 2:51-52

Idolatry and witchcraft were ways of Fir'aun and his people and you were determined to keep those ways with you despite Allah, The Most High, giving you the beautiful religion of Islam. You took these ways with you across the world practicing Voodoo, Juju, Hoodoo and other forms of witchcraft. Your enemy has filled your heart with false hopes in "The American Dream", Democracy, and has imparted in your souls the beauty of false religions through the propagation of holidays like Christmas and Easter. It is so unfortunate that even some who claim to be Muslim hang lights and put-up trees to partake in these festivities. When the Children of Israel took the calf for worship, they placed their gold into a fire in order to create it (the calf). Today, you descendants of the Twelve Tribes, sacrifice each other through killing and oppression, and your youth now hang the golden idols around their necks all for a chance at this "American Dream"!

Those of you in polytheistic religions, you must know that the Roman Catholic Church, the same church who helped to promote the Eugenics movement throughout the world, was also responsible for creating your religion. **It was the Council of Nicea, propagated by the Roman Catholic Church, who were responsible for the creation of the Trinitarian doctrine.** Prophet Isa (Jesus) Prophet Isa never told you to worship him, and he will reject your worship on The Day of Judgement. Allah, The Exalted, says in The Qur'an;

يَٰٓأَهْلَ ٱلْكِتَٰبِ لَا تَغْلُوا۟ فِى دِينِكُمْ وَلَا تَقُولُوا۟ عَلَى ٱللَّهِ إِلَّا ٱلْحَقَّ ۚ إِنَّمَا ٱلْمَسِيحُ عِيسَى ٱبْنُ مَرْيَمَ رَسُولُ ٱللَّهِ وَكَلِمَتُهُۥٓ أَلْقَىٰهَآ إِلَىٰ مَرْيَمَ وَرُوحٌ مِّنْهُ ۖ فَـَٔامِنُوا۟ بِٱللَّهِ وَرُسُلِهِۦ ۖ وَلَا تَقُولُوا۟ ثَلَٰثَةٌ ۚ ٱنتَهُوا۟ خَيْرًا لَّكُمْ ۚ إِنَّمَا ٱللَّهُ إِلَٰهٌ وَٰحِدٌ ۖ سُبْحَٰنَهُۥٓ أَن يَكُونَ لَهُۥ وَلَدٌ ۘ لَّهُۥ مَا فِى ٱلسَّمَٰوَٰتِ وَمَا فِى ٱلْأَرْضِ ۗ وَكَفَىٰ بِٱللَّهِ وَكِيلًا

"O people of the Scripture (Christians)! Do not exceed the limits of your religion, nor say of Allah anything but the truth. The Messiah, Isa (Jesus), son of Maryam (Mary), was (no more than) a Messenger of Allah and His Word, ("Be – and he was) which He bestowed on Maryam (Mary) and a spirit (Ruh) created by Him; so believe in Allah and His Messengers. Say not: "Three (trinity)! Cease! (it is) better for you. For Allah is (the only) One Illah (God), glorified is

He (Far Exalted is He) above having a son. To Him belongs all that is in the heavens and all that is in the earth. And Allah is All-Sufficient as a Disposer of affairs."

Surah An-Nisa, 4:171

All of Allah's Messengers called to the same thing – Tawheed (monotheism, the belief in one God). They also came with scripture which laid down rules and verdicts which the believers should govern themselves by. When these Messengers came, some people believed and some people disbelieved, while others were hypocrites- saying they believed but acted contrary to their supposed convictions. This is true of The Children of Israel, some of them believed and entered into Islam completely, while some of them found entering into Islam difficult and they constantly broke their covenant with Allah, The Exalted and His Messengers. Allah The Exalted, says in The Qur'an;

وَإِذْ أَخَذْنَا مِيثَـٰقَ بَنِىٓ إِسْرَٰٓءِيلَ لَا تَعْبُدُونَ إِلَّا ٱللَّهَ وَبِٱلْوَٰلِدَيْنِ إِحْسَانًا وَذِى ٱلْقُرْبَىٰ
وَٱلْيَتَـٰمَىٰ وَٱلْمَسَـٰكِينِ وَقُولُوا۟ لِلنَّاسِ حُسْنًا وَأَقِيمُوا۟ ٱلصَّلَوٰةَ وَءَاتُوا۟ ٱلزَّكَوٰةَ ثُمَّ تَوَلَّيْتُمْ إِلَّا قَلِيلًا
مِّنكُمْ وَأَنتُم مُّعْرِضُونَ

وَإِذْ أَخَذْنَا مِيثَـٰقَكُمْ لَا تَسْفِكُونَ دِمَآءَكُمْ وَلَا تُخْرِجُونَ أَنفُسَكُم مِّن دِيَـٰرِكُمْ ثُمَّ أَقْرَرْتُمْ
وَأَنتُمْ تَشْهَدُونَ

ثُمَّ أَنتُمْ هَـٰٓؤُلَآءِ تَقْتُلُونَ أَنفُسَكُمْ وَتُخْرِجُونَ فَرِيقًا مِّنكُم مِّن دِيَـٰرِهِمْ تَظَـٰهَرُونَ عَلَيْهِم
بِٱلْإِثْمِ وَٱلْعُدْوَٰنِ وَإِن يَأْتُوكُمْ أُسَـٰرَىٰ تَفْدُوهُمْ وَهُوَ مُحَرَّمٌ عَلَيْكُمْ إِخْرَاجُهُمْ ۚ أَفَتُؤْمِنُونَ
بِبَعْضِ ٱلْكِتَـٰبِ وَتَكْفُرُونَ بِبَعْضٍ ۚ فَمَا جَزَآءُ مَن يَفْعَلُ ذَٰلِكَ مِنكُمْ إِلَّا خِزْىٌ فِى ٱلْحَيَوٰةِ
ٱلدُّنْيَا ۖ وَيَوْمَ ٱلْقِيَـٰمَةِ يُرَدُّونَ إِلَىٰٓ أَشَدِّ ٱلْعَذَابِ ۗ وَمَا ٱللَّهُ بِغَـٰفِلٍ عَمَّا تَعْمَلُونَ

"And (remember) when We took a covenant from the Children of Israel, (saying): Worship none but Allah (Alone) and be dutiful and good to parents, and to kindred, and to orphans and to Al-Masakin (the needy), and speak good to people (i.e., enjoin righteousness and forbid evil, and say the truth about Muhammad ﷺ), and perform As-Salat (Iqamat-as-Salat), and give Zakat. Then you slid back, except a few of you, while you are backsliders. And (remember) when We took your covenant (saying): Shed not the blood of your (people), nor turn your own people from their dwellings. Then, (this) you ratified and (to this) you bear witness. After this, it is you who kill one another and drive out a party of you from their homes, assist (their enemies) against them, in sin and transgression. And if they come to you as captives, you ransom them, although their expulsion was forbidden to you. Then do you believe in part of the Scripture and reject the rest? What is the recompense of those who do so among you, except disgrace in the life of this world, and on the Day of Resurrection they shall be consigned to the most grievous torment. And Allah is not unaware of what you do.

Surah Al-Baqarah, 2:83-85

The majority of the Children of Israel have always been contentious against Allah's Laws, breaking his covenant and changing his Holy Books. The abovementioned ayahs were revealed to criticize the tribes of Jews who lived in Al-Madinah during the time of Prophet Muhammad ﷺ however, other tribes from the Children of Israel have broken these commandments in the same way throughout history. Most recently occurring during the African slave trade when many of the decedents from Children of Israel, even some who later converted to Islam, sold their own people to their enemy. In violating Allah's covenant, you made your enemy stronger, selling your own people to work for him, thereby helping him conquer and develop lands that did not belong to him. Now America and Europe, the main instigators behind COVID-19, is a strong enemy to you and all of humanity. Allah, The Exalted, took your covenant and made promises with you that you would be true faithful servants of His and also that you would be true to all of His Messengers including Prophet Muhammad ﷺ;

ٱلَّذِينَ يَتَّبِعُونَ ٱلرَّسُولَ ٱلنَّبِىَّ ٱلْأُمِّىَّ ٱلَّذِى يَجِدُونَهُۥ مَكْتُوبًا عِندَهُمْ فِى ٱلتَّوْرَىٰةِ وَٱلْإِنجِيلِ
يَأْمُرُهُم بِٱلْمَعْرُوفِ وَيَنْهَىٰهُمْ عَنِ ٱلْمُنكَرِ وَيُحِلُّ لَهُمُ ٱلطَّيِّبَٰتِ وَيُحَرِّمُ عَلَيْهِمُ ٱلْخَبَٰٓئِثَ وَيَضَعُ
عَنْهُمْ إِصْرَهُمْ وَٱلْأَغْلَٰلَ ٱلَّتِى كَانَتْ عَلَيْهِمْ ۚ فَٱلَّذِينَ ءَامَنُوا۟ بِهِۦ وَعَزَّرُوهُ وَنَصَرُوهُ وَٱتَّبَعُوا۟
ٱلنُّورَ ٱلَّذِىٓ أُنزِلَ مَعَهُۥٓ ۙ أُو۟لَٰٓئِكَ هُمُ ٱلْمُفْلِحُونَ

"Those who follow the Messenger, the Prophet who can neither read nor write (i.e. Muhammad ﷺ) whom they find written with them in the Taurat (Torah) (Deut, x viii 15) and the Injeel (Gospel) (John xiv, 16) – he commands them for Al-Ma'ruf (i.e. Islamic Monotheism and all that Islam has ordained); and forbids them from Al-Munkar (i.e. disbelief, polytheism of all kinds, and all that Islam has forbidden); he allows them as lawful At-Tayyibat (i.e. all good and lawful as regards to things, deeds, beliefs, persons, foods), and prohibits them as unlawful Al-Khaba'ith (i.e. all evil and unlawful as regards to things, deeds, beliefs, persons and foods) he releases them from their heavy burdens (of Allah's Covenant with the children of Israel), and from the fetters (bindings) that were upon them. So those who believe in him (Muhammad ﷺ), honor him, help him, and follow the light (the Qur'an) which has been sent down with him, it is they who will be successful."

Surah Al-A'raf, 7:157

Due constant turning away from Allah, in the matters of religion, Allah, The Exalted, turned away from you Children of Israel and this is why you are in such a vulnerable and weakened state today as Allah, The Exalted, says in The Qur'an;

وَإِذْ تَأَذَّنَ رَبُّكَ لَيَبْعَثَنَّ عَلَيْهِمْ إِلَىٰ يَوْمِ ٱلْقِيَـٰمَةِ مَن يَسُومُهُمْ سُوٓءَ ٱلْعَذَابِ ۗ إِنَّ رَبَّكَ
لَسَرِيعُ ٱلْعِقَابِ ۖ وَإِنَّهُۥ لَغَفُورٌ رَّحِيمٌ

"And (remember) when your Lord declared that He would certainly keep on sending against them (i.e. the Jews), till the Day of Resurrection, those who would afflict them with a humiliating torment. Verily, your Lord is Quick in Retribution (for the disobedient, wicked) and certainly He is Oft-Forgiving, Most Merciful (for the obedient and those who beg Allah's Forgiveness."

Surah Al-'A'raf, 7:167

O, Children of Israel! Your enemy is upon you! He has his army surrounding you wherever you may be! From every corner of the world, they are situated and have started a mighty attack against you. **Shaytan has inspired your enemy to move quickly against you because you are a threat to the purity of his bloodline as more and more of your men mate with and marry his (White) women.** Shaytan has convinced them that you are a threat to world health, that you are overpopulating the earth, and that you are beyond becoming civilized due to your low IQs and proneness to criminality. The enemy sees you as a lust-filled threat to the world they want their children to inherit.

Prophet Muhammad ﷺ spoke the truth when he said;

"This world is sweet and dazzling, and Allaah has you put in charge of it to see how you will do and what you will do, so beware of this world and beware of women, for the first fitnah (temptation, trial) that befell the Children of Israel was concerning women."

Reported by Muslim, 4925

And this is still your temptation. The crimes you commit against your own women-folk in Africa, India, the Caribbean, South America, Asia, and amongst the Blacks in North America pale in comparison to what your enemy has ever done to them! You fornicate with them though it is a great sin, leave them with the responsibility of raising the children, beat them, rape them, and kill them at alarming rates.

Your chances of survival depend upon your repentance to Allah, The Exalted, and your purifying your Faith. These are your only hopes for defense. Just as your ancestors were led by Prophet Musa عَلَيْهِ ٱلسَّلَامُ in an escape by night, you are now being called upon through the darkness to move. However, the migration will not take place by foot this time. This migration must occur in the spiritual realm. **For your safety and the safety of your offspring you must flee to Allah and move away from the darkness of polytheism to the light of Faith (Islam).** Your enemy has unleashed a weapon that is part of the ghayb (unseen) thus, your counterattack must be the same (the faith in your hearts), it is only then that the help of Allah, The Most High, will arrive. Allah, The Most High, says in The Qur'an;

إِذَا جَآءَ نَصْرُ ٱللَّهِ وَٱلْفَتْحُ

وَرَأَيْتَ ٱلنَّاسَ يَدْخُلُونَ فِى دِينِ ٱللَّهِ أَفْوَاجًا

فَسَبِّحْ بِحَمْدِ رَبِّكَ وَٱسْتَغْفِرْهُ ۚ إِنَّهُۥ كَانَ تَوَّابًا

"When there comes the Help of Allah and the Conquest. And you see that the people enter Allah's religion (Islam) in crowds. So glorify the Praises of your Lord, and ask His Forgiveness. Verily, He is the One Who Ever accepts the repentance and Who forgives."

Surah An-Nasr, 110:1-3

You are being called upon to discard polytheist beliefs and purify your religion for Allah and Allah alone. Allah, The Most High, says in The Qur'an;

يَـٰٓأَيُّهَا ٱلَّذِينَ ءَامَنُوا۟ ٱدْخُلُوا۟ فِى ٱلسِّلْمِ كَآفَّةً وَلَا تَتَّبِعُوا۟ خُطُوَٰتِ ٱلشَّيْطَـٰنِ ۚ إِنَّهُۥ لَكُمْ عَدُوٌّ
مُّبِينٌ

"O you who believe! Enter perfectly in Islam (by obeying all the rules and regulations of the Islamic religion) and follow not the footsteps of Shaytan (Satan). Verily, he is to you a plain enemy."

Surah Al-Baqarah, 2:208

Allah wishes to forgive you, purify you, and protect you against all harm. Allah, The Exalted, says in The Qur'an;

إِنَّ ٱلَّذِينَ ءَامَنُوا۟ وَٱلَّذِينَ هَادُوا۟ وَٱلنَّصَـٰرَىٰ وَٱلصَّـٰبِـِٔينَ مَنْ ءَامَنَ بِٱللَّهِ وَٱلْيَوْمِ ٱلْـَٔاخِرِ
وَعَمِلَ صَـٰلِحًا فَلَهُمْ أَجْرُهُمْ عِندَ رَبِّهِمْ وَلَا خَوْفٌ عَلَيْهِمْ وَلَا هُمْ يَحْزَنُونَ

"Verily, those who believe and those who are Jews and Christians, and Sabians, whoever believes in Allah and the Last

Day and does righteous good deeds shall have their reward with their Lord, on them shall be no fear, nor shall they grieve.

Surah Al-Baqarah, 2:62

And;

صِبْغَةَ ٱللَّهِۖ وَمَنْ أَحْسَنُ مِنَ ٱللَّهِ صِبْغَةًۖ وَنَحْنُ لَهُۥ عَٰبِدُونَ

"(Our religion ((Islam)) is) the Baptism of Allah: And who can baptize better than Allah? And it is He Whom we worship."

Surah Al-Baqarah, 2:138

O Humanity! Enter into the fold of Islam, where a White person is not considered better than a Black person, nor an Arab considered better than a non-Arab. *Despite you're your enemy says, your affair is not about having "bad genes", it has everything to do with your rebellion towards Allah, The Most High.* Enter into a religion that was created for you by your Lord and is for all of mankind. To enter into this beautiful brotherhood and sisterhood one must take Shahada, that is, they must utter these words;

"I bear witness that there is no God but Allah alone, and that Prophet Muhammad ﷺ is His last and final messenger."

Further, you must start Salat, that is to enjoin the prayer 5 times per day. After that you must pay Zakat, that is give in charity. You must be diligent in seeking knowledge and the first knowledge you should acquire along with learning to pray is the matter of Tawheed. Understanding what the belief in Allah alone means will allow you to discard your previous lifestyles of polytheism and worship Allah completely.

You should beware of whom you take Islamic knowledge from as there are many groups who have diluted this beautiful religion by indulging in polytheistic behaviors. They say that they believe but in truth they are either ignorant or hypocrites and you must not attempt to learn your religion from them. There is one group from amongst the Ummah (community of Muslims) who are best suited for teaching Islam the way that Allah, The Exalted, intended. This group represents Ahlus Sunnah wal Jamaah and they teach the religion of Islam according to the methodology of the Salaf (righteous predecessors) and further may be identified as Salafiyyah. Allah, The Exalted, says about them in The Qur'an;

وَٱعْتَصِمُوا۟ بِحَبْلِ ٱللَّهِ جَمِيعًا وَلَا تَفَرَّقُوا۟ ۚ وَٱذْكُرُوا۟ نِعْمَتَ ٱللَّهِ عَلَيْكُمْ إِذْ كُنتُمْ أَعْدَآءً
فَأَلَّفَ بَيْنَ قُلُوبِكُمْ فَأَصْبَحْتُم بِنِعْمَتِهِۦٓ إِخْوَٰنًا وَكُنتُمْ عَلَىٰ شَفَا حُفْرَةٍ مِّنَ ٱلنَّارِ فَأَنقَذَكُم مِّنْهَا ۗ
كَذَٰلِكَ يُبَيِّنُ ٱللَّهُ لَكُمْ ءَايَٰتِهِۦ لَعَلَّكُمْ تَهْتَدُونَ

وَلْتَكُن مِّنكُمْ أُمَّةٌ يَدْعُونَ إِلَى ٱلْخَيْرِ وَيَأْمُرُونَ بِٱلْمَعْرُوفِ وَيَنْهَوْنَ عَنِ ٱلْمُنكَرِ ۚ
وَأُو۟لَٰٓئِكَ هُمُ ٱلْمُفْلِحُونَ

"And hold fast, all of you together, to the Rope of Allah (i.e. this Qur'an), and be not divided amongst yourselves, and remember Allah's Favor on you, for you were enemies one to another but He joined your hearts together, so that, by His

Grace, you became brethren (in Islamic Faith), and you were on the brink of a pit of Fire, and He saved you from it. Thus Allah makes His Ayat (proofs, evidences, verses, lessons, signs, revelations, etc.,) clear to you that you may be guided. **Let there arise out of you a group of people inviting to all that is good (Islam), enjoining Al-Ma'ruf (i.e., Islamic Monotheism and all that Islam orders on to do) and forbidding Al-Munkar (polytheism and disbelief and all that Islam has forbidden). And it is they who are the successful.**

Surah Al 'Imran, 3:103-104

I encourage those who are upon Salafiyyah, and further those who implement the Qur'an and the Sunnah in the way that the Prophet and His companions did, become even more active in dawah and to be kind and patient in teaching the religion. Those Muslims who are guilty of mixing your religion with falsehood must strive to purify your religion by learning from those who are teaching the religion according to the methodology of the Salaf and do not resist them. They are the ones whom Allah has entrusted with knowledge and they are your truest friends who want good for you and so you should not draw sin upon yourselves by annoying them. Aid them and together support the religion of Allah, The Most High, by guiding non-believers to Islam.

May Allah, The Most High, guide and protect you and your family and give us victory over our enemies. Ameen.

#Expose Scientific Racism

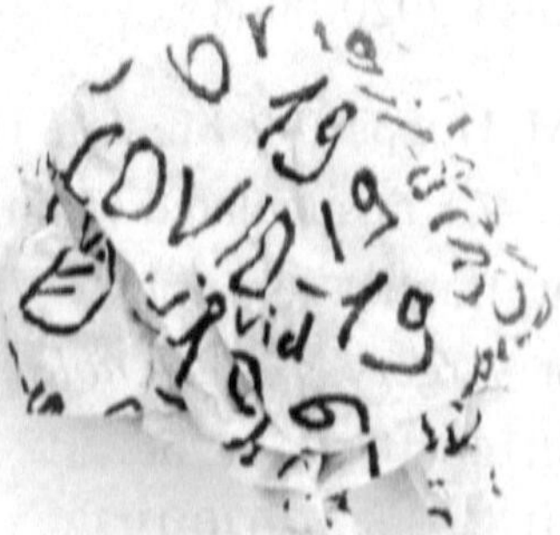

Join the Discussion

There will be many who will not read this book. You can help disseminate the facts. Use the hashtag above and contribute to the discussion.

References for Further Study

Introduction:

1. Chialda, M. Acute Mastoiditis – Beginning of COVID-19 Infection – Case Report. ACTA Medica Transilvanica. December 25(4): 25-27. Doi: 10.2478amtsb-2020-0064

2. Frazier KM, Hooper JE, Mostafa HH, Stewart CM. SARS-CoV-2 Virus Isolated From the Mastoid and Middle Ear: Implications for COVID-19 Precautions During Ear Surgery. *JAMA Otolaryngol Head Neck Surg.* 2020;146(10):964–966. doi:10.1001/jamaoto.2020.1922

3. Vural Fidan, Am J Otolaryngol, https://doi.org/10.1016/j.amjoto.2020.102487

4. Raad N, Ghorbani J, Mikaniki N, Haseli S, Karimi-Galougahi M. Otitis media in coronavirus dis-ease 2019: a case series. J Laryngol Otol. 2021 Jan;135(1):10-13. doi: 10.1017/S0022215120002741. Epub 2021 Jan 7. PMID: 33407978; PMCID: PMC7804088.

5. Kesser BW. News Flash!—SARS-CoV-2 Isolated From the Middle Ear and Mastoid. *JAMA Otolaryngol Head Neck Surg.* 2020;146(10):966–967. doi:10.1001/jamaoto.2020.2067

6. Portin, Petter, and Adam Wilkins. "The Evolving Definition of the Term "Gene"." *Genetics* vol. 205,4 (2017): 1353-1364. doi:10.1534/genetics.116.196956

7. Lawrence, Cera R., "The Eugenics Record Office at Cold Spring Harbor Laboratory (1910-1939)". *Embryo Project Encyclopedia* (2011-04-21). ISSN: 1940-5030 http://embryo.asu.edu/handle/10776/2091

8. Okrent, Daniel. The Guarded Gate (Scribner, 2019).

9. Watson, James D., 1928-. The **Double Helix** : a Personal Account of the Discovery of the Structure **of DNA**. London :Weidenfeld and Nicolson, 1981.

10. Carvalho, Tito,, Zhu, Tian, "The Human Genome Project (1990-2003)". *Embryo Project Encyclopedia* (2014-05-06). ISSN: 1940-5030 http://embryo.asu.edu/handle/10776/7829.

11. New Goals for the U.S. Human Genome Project: 1998-2003. BY FRANCIS S. COLLINS, ARI PATRINOS, ELKE JORDAN, ARAVINDA CHAKRAVARTI, RAYMOND GESTELAND, LEROY WALTERS, THE MEMBERS OF THE DOE AND NIH PLANNING GROUPS. SCIENCE23 OCT 1998 : 682-689.

12. Crystal Structure of a Group I Ribozyme Domain: Principles of RNA Packing BY JAMIE H. CATE, ANNE R. GOODING, ELAINE PODELL, KAIHONG ZHOU, BARBARA L. GOLDEN, CRAIG E. KUNDROT, THOMAS R. CECH, JENNIFER A. DOUDNA. SCIENCE20 SEP 1996 : 1678-1685.

13. Isaacson, Walter. The Code Breaker: Jennifer Doudna, Gene Editing, and the Future of the Human Race. Simon & Schuster. 2021.

14. Cold Spring Harbor Laboratory. "Phage Courses Begin at Cold Spring Harbor". Library & Archives. http://library.cshl.edu/resources/library-newsletter/161-2012-10-newsletter-2/331-phage-courses-begin-at-cold-spring-harbor . Accessed April 18, 2021.

15. Barenkamp SJ, St Geme JW 3rd. Genes encoding high-molecular-weight adhesion proteins of nontypeable Haemophilus influenzae are part of gene clusters. Infect Immun. 1994 Aug;62(8):3320-8. doi: 10.1128/IAI.62.8.3320-3328.1994. PMID: 8039903; PMCID: PMC302962.

Chapter One:

1. Joseph Adrian L Buensalido et al. "Haemophilus Influenzae Infections", Medscape, 2019. https://emedicine.medscape.com/article/218271-overview

2. Sunnan Ibn Majah. Book 36, Hadith 94, https://sunnah.com/ibnmajah/36/94. Accessed 2020.

3. Finer, Lawrence B. "Trends in premarital sex in the United States, 1954-2003." Public health reports (Washington, D.C. : 1974) vol. 122,1 (2007): 73-8. doi:10.1177/003335490712200110

4. "Global Morality". Pew Research Center. 2013. https://www.pewresearch.org/global/interactives/global-morality/

5. The Noble Qur'an. Saheeh International, 1997, https://quran.com/8. Accessed 1 April 2020.

6. Al-Jauziyah, Imam Ibn Qayyim. Healing with the Medicine of the Prophet ﷺ. July 2010 ed., Riyadh, DARUSSALAM, 751 H.

7. Centers for Dis-ease Control, et al. "Plague Symptoms." CDC, 2018, https://www.cdc.gov/plague/symptoms/index.html. Accessed 4 12 2020.

8. Cascella, Marco, et al. "Features, Evaluation, and Treatment Coronavirus (COVID-19)." NCBI Bookshelf, StatPearls Publishing, 2020, https://www.ncbi.nlm.nih.gov/books/NBK554776/. Accessed 22 April 2020.

9. Langereis JD, de Jonge MI. Invasive Dis-ease Caused by Nontypeable Haemophilus influenzae. Emerg Infect Dis. 2015;21(10):1711-1718. https://dx.doi.org/10.3201/eid2110.150004

10. Centers for Dis-ease Control. "People with Certain Medical Conditions." CDC, 1 December 2020, https://www.cdc.gov/coronavirus/2019-ncov/need-extra-precautions/people-with-medical-conditions.html. Accessed 5 December 2020.

11. Langereis, J D., Jonge M L. Invasive Dis-ease Caused by Nontypeable Haemophilus Influenzae. Emerging Infectious Dis-eases Vol. 21, No. 10, October 2015. DOI: http://dx.doi.org/10.3201/eid2110.150004

12. Gulraiz, Fahad, et al. "Haemophilus influenzae increases the susceptibility and inflammatory response of airway epithelia cells to viral infections." The FASEB Journal, no. 29, 2015, pp. 849-858,

www.fasebj.org. Accessed 23 April 2020.

13. Cascella M, Rajnik M, Cuomo A, Dulebohn SC, Di Napoli R. Features, Evaluation, and Treatment of Coronavirus. 2020 Oct 4. In: StatPearls [Internet]. Treasure Island (FL): StatPearls Publishing; 2020 Jan–. PMID: 32150360. Originally accessed April 23, 2020.

14. Wedzicha, J. A. "Rose of viruses in exacerbations of chronic obstructive pulmonary dis-ease." Proceedings of the American Thoracic Society, vol. 1, no. 2, 2006, pp. 115-120.

15. Wilkinson, T M A., et al. "Effect of interactions between lower airway bacterial and rhinoviral infection in exacerbations of COPD." Chest, vol. 129, no. 2, 2006, pp. 317-324.

16. Papi, A., et al. "Infections and airway inflammation in chronic obstructive pulmonary dis-ease severe exacerbations." American Journal of Respiratory and Critical Care Medicine, vol. 173, no. 10, 2006, pp. 1114-1121.

17. King, Paul T., and Roleen Sharma. "The Lung Immune Response to Nontypeable Haemophilus influenzae." Hindawi Publishing Corporation, no. 706376, 2015, p. 14. http://dx.doi.org/10.1155/2015/706376. Accessed 21 April 2020.

18. Turk DC. The pathogenicity of Haemophilus influenzae. J Med Microbiol. 1984 Aug;18(1):1-16. doi: 10.1099/00222615-18-1-1. PMID: 6146721.

19. Bluestone, C. D. Otitis media in children: to treat or

not to treat? N. Engl. J. Med. 306:1399-1404. PubMed.

20. Murphy, T. F., and M. A. Apicella. Nontypeable Haemophilus influenzae: a review of clinical aspects, surface antigens and the human response to infection. Rev. Infect. Dis. 9:1-15, https://pubmed.ncbi.nlm.nih.gov/3547567/.

21. Cevik M, Moncayo-Nieto OL, Evans MJ. Non-typeable Haemophilus influenzae-associated early pregnancy loss: an emerging neonatal and maternal pathogen. Infection. 2020 Apr;48(2):285-288. doi: 10.1007/s15010-019-01359-6. Epub 2019 Sep 23. PMID: 31549360; PMCID: PMC7292808.

22. Szelestey, Blake R., et al. "Haemophilus Responses to Nutritional Immunity: Epigenetic and Morphological Contribution to Biofilm Architecture, Invasion, Persistence, and Dis-ease Severity." PLoS Pathogens, vol. 9, no. 10, 2003. DOI: 10.1371/journal.ppat.1003709.

23. Nationwide Children's Hospital. "Why some ear, respiratory infections become chronic." ScienceDaily. ScienceDaily, 22 November 2013. <www.sciencedaily.com/releases/2013/11/131122103934.htm>

24. Lei J, Kusov Y, Hilgenfeld R. Nsp3 of coronaviruses: Structures and functions of a large multi-domain protein. Antiviral Res. 2018 Jan; 149:58-74 [PubMed: 29128390]

25. Amraei, Razie, and Nader Rahimi. "COVID-19, Renin-Angiotensin System and Endothelial

Dysfunction." Cells vol. 9,7 1652. 9 Jul. 2020, doi:10.3390/cells9071652

26. McCance, Kathryn L., et al. Pathophysiology The Biologic Basis for Dis-ease in Adults and Children. Seventh ed., St. Louis, Elsevier Mosby, 2014. P. 192

27. Clementi, C. F., and T. F. Murphy. "Non-typeable Haemophilus influenzae invasion and persistence in the human respiratory tract." Frontiers in Cellular and Infection Microbiology, vol. 1, no. 1, 2011.

28. Kerr JR. Cell adhesion molecules in the pathogenesis of and host defence against microbial infection. Mol Pathol. 1999 Aug;52(4):220-30. doi: 10.1136/mp.52.4.220. PMID: 10694943; PMCID: PMC395703.

29. Tong, Ming et al. "Elevated Expression of Serum Endothelial Cell Adhesion Molecules in COVID-19 Patients." The Journal of infectious dis-eases vol. 222,6 (2020): 894-898. doi:10.1093/infdis/jiaa349

30. Jono, H., and T. Shuto. "Transforming growth factor B-Smad signaling pathway cooperates with NF-kB to mediate nontypeable Haemophilus influenzae-induced MUC2 mucin transcription." Journal of Biological Chemistry,, vol. 277, no. 47, 2002, pp. 44547-45557.

31. Khair, O. A., et al. "Bacterial induced release of inflammatory mediators by bronchial epithelial cells." European Respiratory Journal, vol. 9, no. 9, 1996, pp. 1913-1922.

32. Dupin, Nicolas, et al. Distribution of human

herpesvirus-8 latently infected cells in Kaposi's sarcoma, multicentric Castleman's dis-ease, and primary effusion lymphoma. Proceedings of the National Academy of Sciences Apr 1999, 96 (8) 4546-4551; DOI: 10.1073/pnas.96.8.4546.

33. Mackow ER, Gavrilovskaya IN. Hantavirus regulation of endothelial cell functions. Thromb Haemost. 2009 Dec;102(6):1030-41. doi: 10.1160/TH09-09-0640. PMID: 19967132.

34. Sajjan, U. S., et al. "H. influenzae potentiates airway epithelial cell responses to rhinovirus by increasing ICAM-1 and TLR3 expression." FASEB J., vol. 20, 2006, pp. 2121-2123.

35. NCBI. "Entrez Gene: intercellular adhesion molecule 1." https://www.ncbi.nlm.nih.gov/gene?Db=gene&Cmd=DetailsSearch&Term=3383#bibliography

36. Nguyen, Lily P., et al. "Similar allergic inflammation in the middle ear and the upper airway: Evidence linking otitis media with effusion to the united airways concept." American Academy of Allergy, Asthma, and Immunology, 2004. doi:10.1016/j.jaci.2004.07.061.

37. Wu, Z.; McGoogan, J.M. Characteristics of and Important Lessons from the Coronavirus Dis-ease 2019 (COVID-19) Outbreak in China: Summary of a Report of 72 314 Cases From the Chinese Center for Dis-ease Control and Prevention. JAMA 2020, 323, 1239-1242.

38. Mehlotra, Rajeev K. "Chemokine receptor gene

polymorphisms and COVID-19: Could knowledge gained from HIV/AIDS be important?." Infection, genetics and evolution : journal of molecular epidemiology and evolutionary genetics in infectious dis-eases vol. 85 (2020): 104512. doi:10.1016/j.meegid.2020.104512

39. P. Galea, C. Vermot-Desroches, C. Le Contel, J. Wijdenes, J.-C. Chermann. Circulating cell adhesion molecules in HIV1-infected patients as indicator markers for AIDS progression, Research in Immunology, Volume 148, Issue 2, 1997, Pages 109-117, ISSN 0923-2494, https://doi.org/10.1016/S0923-2494(97)82482-0.

40. Tardif, Mélanie R, and Michel J Tremblay. "Presence of host ICAM-1 in human immunodeficiency virus type 1 virions increases productive infection of CD4+ T lymphocytes by favoring cytosolic delivery of viral material." Journal of virology vol. 77,22 (2003): 12299-309. doi:10.1128/jvi.77.22.12299-12309.2003

41. Raja, Aarti et al. "CD4 binding site antibodies inhibit human immunodeficiency virus gp120 envelope glycoprotein interaction with CCR5." Journal of virology vol. 77,1 (2003): 713-8. doi:10.1128/jvi.77.1.713-718.2003

42. Puigdomènech I, Massanella M, Izquierdo-Useros N, Ruiz-Hernandez R, Curriu M, Bofill M, Martinez-Picado J, Juan M, Clotet B, Blanco J. HIV transfer between CD4 T cells does not require LFA-1 binding to ICAM-1 and is governed by the interaction of HIV envelope glycoprotein with CD4. Retrovirology. 2008

Mar 31;5:32. doi: 10.1186/1742-4690-5-32. PMID: 18377648; PMCID: PMC2359761

43. Allen, A.G., Chung, C.H., Atkins, A., et al., 2018. Gene editing of HIV-1 co-receptors to prevent and/or cure virus infection. Front Microbiol. 9, 2940.

44. Xu, M.M., 2020. CCR5-delta32 biology, gene editing, and warnings for the future of CRISPR-Cas9 as a human and humane gene editing tool. Cell Biosci. 10,48.

45. Mehlotra, Rajeev K. "Chemokine receptor gene polymorphisms and COVID-19: Could knowledge gained from HIV/AIDS be important?." Infection, genetics and evolution : journal of molecular epidemiology and evolutionary genetics in infectious dis-eases vol. 85 (2020): 104512. doi:10.1016/j.meegid.2020.104512

46. Collins LF, Havers FP, Tunali A, Thomas S, Clennon JA, Wiley Z, Tobin-D'Angelo M, Parrott T, Read TD, Satola SW, Petit RA 3rd, Farley MM. Invasive Nontypeable Haemophilus influenzae Infection Among Adults With HIV in Metropolitan Atlanta, Georgia, 2008-2018. JAMA. 2019 Dec 24;322(24):2399-2410. doi: 10.1001/jama.2019.18800. PMID: 31860046; PMCID: PMC6990662.

47. Hioe CE, Tuen M, Vasiliver-Shamis G, Alvarez Y, Prins KC, Banerjee S, et al. (2011) HIV Envelope gp120 Activates LFA-1 on CD4 T-Lymphocytes and Increases Cell Susceptibility to LFA-1-Targeting Leukotoxin (LtxA). PLoS ONE 6(8): e23202.

https://doi.org/10.1371/journal.pone.0023202

48. Kaur, Manpreet, and Scott C Kachlany. "Aggregatibacter actinomycetemcomitans leukotoxin (LtxA; Leukothera) induces cofilin dephosphorylation and actin depolymerization during killing of malignant monocytes." Microbiology (Reading, England) vol. 160,Pt 11 (2014): 2443-2452. doi:10.1099/mic.0.082347-0

49. Nørskov-Lauritsen, Niels. "Classification, identification, and clinical significance of Haemophilus and Aggregatibacter species with host specificity for humans." Clinical microbiology reviews vol. 27,2 (2014): 214-40. doi:10.1128/CMR.00103-13

50. Slots, J et al. "Actinobacillus actinomycetemcomitans in human periodontal dis-ease: a cross-sectional microbiological investigation." Infection and immunity vol. 29,3 (1980): 1013-20.

51. DiFranco K. M., Gupta A., Galusha L. E., Perez J., Nguyen T. V., Fineza C. D., Kachlany S. C. (2012). Leukotoxin (Leukothera®) targets active leukocyte function antigen-1 (LFA-1) protein and triggers a lysosomal mediated cell death pathway. J Biol Chem 287, 17618–17627. 10.1074/jbc.M111.314674

52. Hioe C. E., Tuen M., Vasiliver-Shamis G., Alvarez Y., Prins K. C., Banerjee S., Nádas A., Cho M. W., Dustin M. L., Kachlany S. C. (2011). HIV envelope gp120 activates LFA-1 on CD4 T-lymphocytes and increases cell susceptibility to LFA-1-targeting leukotoxin (LtxA). PLoS ONE 6, e23202.

10.1371/journal.pone.0023202

53. Stenderup K., Rosada C., Dam T. N., Salerno E., Belinka B. A., Kachlany S. C. (2011). Resolution of psoriasis by a leukocyte-targeting bacterial protein in a humanized mouse model. J Invest Dermatol 131, 2033–2039. 10.1038/jid.2011.161

54. Korostoff J., Wang J. F., Kieba I., Miller M., Shenker B. J., Lally E. T. (1998). Actinobacillus actinomycetemcomitans leukotoxin induces apoptosis in HL-60 cells. Infect Immun 66, 4474–4483.

55. Korostoff J., Yamaguchi N., Miller M., Kieba I., Lally E. T. (2000). Perturbation of mitochondrial structure and function plays a central role in Actinobacillus actinomycetemcomitans leukotoxin-induced apoptosis. Microb Pathog 29, 267–278. 10.1006/mpat.2000.0390

56. Sunan Ibn Majah. Volume 4. Book 29, Hadith 3349.

57. Santonicola, Antonella et al. "Eating Disorders and Gastrointestinal Dis-eases." Nutrients vol. 11,12 3038. 12 Dec. 2019, doi:10.3390/nu11123038

58. Godfred-Cato S, Bryant B, Leung J, et al. COVID-19–Associated Multisystem Inflammatory Syndrome in Children — United States, March–July 2020. MMWR Morb Mortal Wkly Rep 2020;69:1074–1080. DOI: http://dx.doi.org/10.15585/mmwr.mm6932e2external icon

59. Antoni, Lena et al. "Intestinal barrier in inflammatory bowel dis-ease." World journal of gastroenterology vol. 20,5 (2014): 1165-79.

doi:10.3748/wjg.v20.i5.1165

60. Giron, L. B., et al., Severe COVID-19 Is Fueled by Disrupted Gut Barrier Integrity

61. medRxiv 2020.11.13.20231209; doi: https://doi.org/10.1101/2020.11.13.20231209

62. Scott, David W et al. "Identification of a high-mannose ICAM-1 glycoform: effects of ICAM-1 hypoglycosylation on monocyte adhesion and outside in signaling." American journal of physiology. Cell physiology vol. 305,2 (2013): C228-37. doi:10.1152/ajpcell.00116.201

63. Vainer B, Nielsen OH. Changed colonic profile of P-selectin, platelet-endothelial cell adhesion molecule-1 (PECAM-1), intercellular adhesion molecule-1 (ICAM-1), ICAM-2, and ICAM-3 in inflammatory bowel dis-ease. Clin Exp Immunol. 2000 Aug;121(2):242-7. doi: 10.1046/j.1365-2249.2000.01296.x. PMID: 10931137; PMCID: PMC1905699.

64. McCance, K. L., & Huether, S. E. (2010). Pathophysiology: The biologic basis for dis-ease in adults and children (6th ed.) p. 194.

65. Black, Jacquelyn G, and Laura J. Black. Microbiology: Principles and Explorations. Hoboken, NJ: John Wiley & Sons, Inc, 2008. Print. P. 342.

66. Centers for Dis-ease Control. Antibiotic Resistance Threats Report 2019, https://www.cdc.gov/drugresistance/biggest-

threats.html

67. G.F. Kroker, "Chronic Candidiasis and Allergy", in Brostoff and S.J. Challacombe, eds., Food Allergy and Intolerance (Philadelphia: W.B. Saunders, 1987, 850-72.

68. Delaloye, Julie, and Thierry Calandra. "Invasive candidiasis as a cause of sepsis in the critically ill patient." Virulence vol. 5,1 (2014): 161-9. doi:10.4161/viru.26187

69. Song, Ge et al. "Fungal Co-infections Associated with Global COVID-19 Pandemic: A Clinical and Diagnostic Perspective from China." Mycopathologia vol. 185,4 (2020): 599-606. doi:10.1007/s11046-020-00462-9

70. Amorim Dos Santos, Juliana et al. "Oral mucosal lesions in a COVID-19 patient: New signs or secondary manifestations?." International journal of infectious dis-eases : IJID : official publication of the International Society for Infectious Dis-eases vol. 97 (2020): 326-328. doi:10.1016/j.ijid.2020.06.012

71. Todd, R M, and N V O'Donohoe. "Acute acquired haemolytic anaemia associated with herpes simplex infection." Archives of dis-ease in childhood vol. 33,172 (1958): 524-6. doi:10.1136/adc.33.172.524

72. National Institutes of Health. "Hemolytic Anemia" https://www.nhlbi.nih.gov/health-topics/hemolytic-anemia

73. Van Dijk W, Mackiewicz A. Interleukin-6-type

cytokine-induced changes in acute phase protein glycosylation. Ann N Y Acad Sci. 1995 Jul 21;762:319-30. doi: 10.1111/j.1749-6632.1995.tb32336.x. PMID: 7545370.

74. Dewald, Justine H et al. "Role of Cytokine-Induced Glycosylation Changes in Regulating Cell Interactions and Cell Signaling in Inflammatory Dis-eases and Cancer." Cells vol. 5,4 43. 29 Nov. 2016, doi:10.3390/cells5040043

75. Godfred-Cato S, Bryant B, Leung J, et al. COVID-19–Associated Multisystem Inflammatory Syndrome in Children — United States, March–July 2020. MMWR Morb Mortal Wkly Rep 2020;69:1074–1080. DOI: http://dx.doi.org/10.15585/mmwr.mm6932e2external icon

76. Joseph Adrian L Buensalido et al. "Haemophilus Influenzae Infections", Medscape, 2019. https://emedicine.medscape.com/article/218271-overview

77. Arroyo-Mendoza, Melissa et al. "Effect of testosterone and estrogen supplementation on the resistance to systemic Candida albicans infection in mice." Heliyon vol. 6,7 e04437. 12 Jul. 2020, doi:10.1016/j.heliyon.2020.e04437

78. US Department of Health and Human Services/Centers for Dis-ease Control and Prevention. "Disparities in Incidence of COVID-19 Among Underrepresented Racial/Ethnic Groups in Counties Identified as Hotspots During June 5–18, 2020 — 22 States,

February–June 2020." Morbidity and Mortality Weekly Report, CDC, 21 August 2020, https://www.cdc.gov/mmwr/volumes/69/wr/mm6933e1.htm. Accessed 5 December 2020.

79. Le, Chi Huu Hong. "The Prevalence of Anemia and Moderate-Severe Anemia in the US Population (NHANES 2003-2012)." PloS one vol. 11,11 e0166635. 15 Nov. 2016, doi:10.1371/journal.pone.0166635

80. Trattler Ross, Jones Adrian. "Better Health through Natural Healing". Hinkler Books Pty Ltd; 2nd edition (October 1, 2004). P. 67-68

81. Klein, Joshua S et al. "A dimeric form of the HIV-1 antibody 2G12 elicits potent antibody-dependent cellular cytotoxicity." AIDS (London, England) vol. 24,11 (2010): 1633-40. doi:10.1097/qad.0b013e32833ad8c8

82. Zitzmann N, Block T, Methta A, Rudd P, Burton D, Wilson I, Platt F, Butters T, Dwek RA. Glycosylation: dis-ease targets and therapy. Adv Exp Med Biol. 2005;564:1-2. doi: 10.1007/0-387-25515-X_1. PMID: 16400797.

83. Platt EJ, Gomes MM, Kabat D. Kinetic mechanism for HIV-1 neutralization by antibody 2G12 entails reversible glycan binding that slows cell entry. Proc Natl Acad Sci U S A. 2012 May 15;109(20):7829-34. doi: 10.1073/pnas.1109728109. Epub 2012 Apr 30. PMID: 22547820; PMCID: PMC3356642.

84. Mao QQ, Ip SP, Xian YF, Hu Z, Che CT.

Antidepressant-like effect of peony: a mini-review. Pharm Biol. 2012 Jan;50(1):72-7. doi: 10.3109/13880209.2011.602696. PMID: 22196583.

85. Marafini, Irene, and Giovanni Monteleone. "Therapeutic Oligonucleotides for Patients with Inflammatory Bowel Dis-eases." Biologics : targets & therapy vol. 14 47-51. 15 Jun. 2020, doi:10.2147/BTT.S257638

86. Walter Reinisch, Kenneth Hung, Mina Hassan-Zahraee, Fabio Cataldi, Targeting Endothelial Ligands: ICAM-1/alicaforsen, MAdCAM-1, Journal of Crohn's and Colitis, Volume 12, Issue suppl_2, August 2018, Pages S669–S677, https://doi.org/10.1093/ecco-jcc/jjy059

87. Martinez-Lopez, Nuria et al. "System-wide Benefits of Intermeal Fasting by Autophagy." Cell metabolism vol. 26,6 (2017): 856-871.e5. doi:10.1016/j.cmet.2017.09.020

88. Hayflick L: Biological aging is no longer an unsolved problem, Ann N Y Acad Sci 1100:1-13, 2007. Review.

89. Gassen, N. C., Jan, P., Thomas, B., Frederik, D., Jackson, E., Katja, W., Marcel, A. M. (2020). Analysis of SARS-CoV-2 controlled autophagy reveals spermidine, MK-2206, and niclosamide as putative antiviral therapeutics. bioRxiv, 04(15), 997254. https://doi.org/10.1101/2020. 04.15.997254

90. Martinez-Lopez, Nuria et al. "System-wide Benefits of Intermeal Fasting by Autophagy." Cell metabolism

vol. 26,6 (2017): 856-871.e5. doi:10.1016/j.cmet.2017.09.020

91. Moussa, Ahmed et al. "Antifungal activity of four honeys of different types from Algeria against pathogenic yeast: Candida albicans and Rhodotorula sp." Asian Pacific journal of tropical biomedicine vol. 2,7 (2012): 554-7. doi:10.1016/S2221-1691(12)60096-3

92. Ndiaye, Mary et al. "The grape antioxidant resveratrol for skin disorders: promise, prospects, and challenges." Archives of biochemistry and biophysics vol. 508,2 (2011): 164-70. doi:10.1016/j.abb.2010.12.030

93. Adhami, Vaqar Mustafa et al. "Cancer chemoprevention by pomegranate: laboratory and clinical evidence." Nutrition and cancer vol. 61,6 (2009): 811-5. doi:10.1080/01635580903285064

94. Lakhan, Ram et al. "Prevalence of Depression, Anxiety, and Stress during COVID-19 Pandemic." Journal of neurosciences in rural practice vol. 11,4 (2020): 519-525. doi:10.1055/s-0040-1716442

95. Walsh, Kathleen Marie et al. "Effects of a Mindfulness Meditation App on Subjective Well-Being: Active Randomized Controlled Trial and Experience Sampling Study." JMIR mental health vol. 6,1 e10844. 8 Jan. 2019, doi:10.2196/10844

96. Mostafa HH, Fissel JA, Fanelli B, Bergman Y, Gniazdowski V, Dadlani M, Carroll KC, Colwell RR, Simner PJ. 2020. Metagenomic next-generation sequencing of nasopharyngeal specimens collected

from confirmed and suspect COVID-19 patients. mBio 11:e01969-20. https://doi.org/10.1128/ mBio.01969-20.

97. Xiaojuan Zhu, Yiyue Ge, Tao Wu, Kangchen Zhao, Yin Chen, Bin Wu, Fengcai Zhu, Baoli Zhu, Lunbiao Cui, Co-infection with respiratory pathogens among COVID-2019 cases, Virus Research, Volume 285, 2020, 198005, ISSN 0168-1702, https://doi.org/10.1016/j.virusres.2020.198005

98. Louise Lansbury, Benjamin Lim, Vadsala Baskaran, Wei Shen Lim, Co-infections in people with COVID-19: a systematic review and meta-analysis, Journal of Infection, Volume 81, Issue 2, 2020, Pages 266-275, ISSN 0163-4453, https://doi.org/10.1016/j.jinf.2020.05.046

Chapter Two:

1. "Same-Sex Marriage Around the World." Pew Research Center, Washington, D.C. (October 28, 2019) https://www.pewforum.org/fact-sheet/gay-marriage-around-the-world/

2. U.S. News & World Report. Best Countries Overall Rankings 2021. https://www.usnews.com/media/best-countries/overall-rankings-2021.pdf Accessed: April 21, 2021.

3. Centers for Disease Control. Reported STDs Reach All-time High for 6th Consecutive Year. April 13, 2021.

https://www.cdc.gov/media/releases/2021/p0413-stds.html Accessed: April 21, 2021.

4. U.S. Department of Health and Human Services. 2020. Sexually Transmitted Infections National Strategic Plan for the United States: 2021–2025. Washington, DC.

5. Ingraham NR. The value of penicillin alone in the prevention and treatment of congenital syphilis. *Acta Derm Venereol*. 1951;31(Suppl 24):60–88.

6. "The Rise of Asian Americans." Pew Research Center, Washington, D.C. (April 4, 2013). https://www.pewresearch.org/social-trends/2012/06/19/the-rise-of-asian-americans/

7. "Intermarriage in the U.S. 50 Years After Loving v. Virginia." Pew Research Center, Washington, D.C. (May 18, 2017) https://www.pewresearch.org/social-trends/2017/05/18/intermarriage-in-the-u-s-50-years-after-loving-v-virginia/

8. "The rise of multiracial and multiethnic babies in the U.S." Pew Research Center, Washington, D.C. (June 6, 2017). https://www.pewresearch.org/fact-tank/2017/06/06/the-rise-of-multiracial-and-multiethnic-babies-in-the-u-s/

9. "Among U.S. cohabiters, 18% have a partner of a different race or ethnicity." Pew Research Center, Washington, D.C. (June 8, 2017) https://www.pewresearch.org/fact-tank/2017/06/08/among-u-s-cohabiters-18-have-a-partner-of-a-different-race-or-ethnicity/

10. "LGBT Identification Rises to 5.6% in Latest U.S. Estimate." Gallop Poll. (February 24, 2021) https://news.gallup.com/poll/329708/lgbt-identification-rises-latest-estimate.aspx

11. "Bisexual adults are far less likely than gay men and lesbians to be 'out' to the people in their lives." Pew Research Center, Washington, D.C. (June 18, 2019). https://www.pewresearch.org/fact-tank/2019/06/18/bisexual-adults-are-far-less-likely-than-gay-men-and-lesbians-to-be-out-to-the-people-in-their-lives/

12. U.S. Centers for Disease Control. The Tuskegee Timeline. https://www.cdc.gov/tuskegee/timeline.htm . Washington, D.C. Accessed: April 21, 2021.

13. U.S. Department of Health & Human Services. HHS Organizational Chart. Washington, D.C. https://www.hhs.gov/about/agencies/orgchart/index.html?language=en Accessed: April 21, 2021.

Chapter Three:

1. "Eugenics". *Unified Medical Language System (Psychological Index Terms)*. Bethesda, Maryland: National Library of Medicine. 2009.

2. "Eugenics". Stanford Encyclopedia of Philosophy. Center for the Study of Language and Information, Stanford University. 2 July 2014.

3. Kingman, D. Ancient Sparta – a perfect gerontocracy? Intergenerational Foundation. 5th February 2017.

Accessed 14th April 2021.

4. Darwin, Charles, 1809-1882. On The Origin of Species by Means of Natural Selection, or Preservation of Favoured Races in the Struggle for Life. London :John Murray, 1859.

5. *Francis Galton. The American Journal of Sociology. Volume X; July, 1904; No. 1*

Chapter Four

1. "Eugenics courses taught in UR biology department in mid-1900s." The Collegian, The University of Richmond. Richmond, Virginia. 23 April 2021. https://www.thecollegianur.com/article/2021/04/eugenics-courses-taught-in-biology-department-for-43-years

2. EUGENICS IN THE COLLEGES. Journal of Heredity, Volume 5, Issue 4, April 1914, Page 186, https://doi.org/10.1093/oxfordjournals.jhered.a107837

3. The Cult of Quality: White Eugenics and Black Responses in the United States, 1900-1934. March 2015USURJ University of Saskatchewan Undergraduate Research Journal 1(2) DOI: 10.32396/usurj.v1i2.80

4. W.E.B. Du Bois, "The Talented Tenth," from The Negro Problem: A Series of Articles by Representative Negroes of To-day (New York, 1903).

5. Du Bois, W. E. B. (William Edward Burghardt), 1868-1963. Black folk and birth control, ca. June 1932. W.

E. B. Du Bois Papers (MS 312). Special Collections and University Archives, University of Massachusetts Amherst Libraries

6. Britannica, The Editors of Encyclopedia. "Margaret Sanger". Encyclopedia Britannica, 10 Sep. 2020, https://www.britannica.com/biography/Margaret-Sanger. Accessed 27 April 2021.

7. "What Margaret Sanger Really Said About Eugenics and Race." Time Magazine. 14, October 2016. https://time.com/4081760/margaret-sanger-history-eugenics/

8. Bedford R. Heredity As Ideology: Ideas of the Woman's Christian Temperance Union of The United States and Ontario on Heredity and Social Reform, 1880-1910. Can Bull Med Hist. 2015 Spring;32(1):77-100. doi: 10.3138/cbmh.32.1.77. PMID: 28155455.

9. Deenesh Sohoni. "Unsuitable Suitors: Anti-Miscegenation Laws, Naturalization Laws, and the Construction of Asian Identities." *Law & Society Review*, vol. 41, no. 3, 2007, pp. 587–618. *JSTOR*, www.jstor.org/stable/4623396. Accessed 28 Apr. 2021.

10. Odijie, Michael (2018). "The Fear of 'Yellow Peril' and the Emergence of European Federalist Movement". The International History Review. 40 (2): 359.

11. Marchetti, Gina (1994). Romance and the "Yellow Peril": Race, Sex, and Discursive Strategies in Hollywood Fiction. University of California Press. ISBN 9780520914629.

12. Richard Jaccoma (1978). "Yellow Peril": The Adventures of Sir John Weymouth-Smythe: a Novel. Richard Marek Publishers. ISBN 0-399-90007-1.

13. Stoneman, Rod (8 November 2014). "Far East Fu fighting: The Yellow Peril – Dr Fu Manchu and the Rise of Chinophobia". The Irish Times. Archived from the original on 19 January 2015. Retrieved 4 January 2015.

14. Cold Spring Harbor Library. "Eugenics Record Office" Archives. https://library.cshl.edu/special-collections/eugenics Access date: 24, April, 2021.

15. Gur-Arie, Rachel, "Harry Hamilton Laughlin (1880-1943)". Embryo Project Encyclopedia (2014-12-19). ISSN: 1940-5030 http://embryo.asu.edu/handle/10776/8271.

16. "Henry H. Laughlin Biography. Truman State University. http://library.truman.edu/manuscripts/laughlinbio.asp Accessed: 27, April, 2021.

17. "Racial and Ethnic Disparities Continue in Pregnancy-Related Deaths." Centers for Disease Control. September 5, 2019. https://www.cdc.gov/media/releases/2019/p0905-racial-ethnic-disparities-pregnancy-deaths.html

18. McGuire, Thomas G, and Jeanne Miranda. "New evidence regarding racial and ethnic disparities in mental health: policy implications." Health affairs (Project Hope) vol. 27,2 (2008): 393-403. doi:10.1377/hlthaff.27.2.393

19. Barlett, Donald L.; Steele, James B. (13 May 2003). "The Oily Americans". Time. Retrieved 8 July 2008.

20. "CIW Department of Genetics". Cold Spring Harbor Library. https://library.cshl.edu/special-collections/carnegie-institution-of-washington Accessed: 28, April, 2021.

21. "Albert Blakeslee 1874-1954". Carnegie Institution for Science. https://dpb.carnegiescience.edu/history/carnegie-figures/albert-blakeslee-1874-1954 Accessed 29, April, 2021.

22. Glass, Bently. "Milislav Demerec 1895-1966: A Biographical Memoir". National Academy of Sciences. Washington, D.C. (1971). http://www.nasonline.org/publications/biographical-memoirs/memoir-pdfs/demerec-milislav.pdf

23. University Of Liverpool. "Biologists Discover Why 10 Percent Of Europeans Are Safe From HIV Infection." ScienceDaily. ScienceDaily, 3 April 2005. <www.sciencedaily.com/releases/2005/03/050325234239.htm>.

24. Peter Bendzko and Hans Joos. Issued: April 21, 2011. "Stale Lysis Buffer Mixture for Extracting Nucleic Acids". Patent No.: US 2011/009687 A1. United States Patent and Trademark Office. https://patents.google.com/patent/US20110092687A1/en

25. Ute V. Solloch, Kathrin Lang, Vinzenz Lange, Irina Böhme, Alexander H. Schmidt, Jürgen Sauter.

Frequencies of gene variant CCR5-Δ32 in 87 countries based on next-generation sequencing of 1.3 million individuals sampled from 3 national DKMS donor centers. Human Immunology, Volume 78, Issues 11–12, 2017, Pages 710-717, ISSN 0198-8859, https://doi.org/10.1016/j.humimm.2017.10.001.

26. "1944: DNA is Transforming Principle". National Human Genome Research Institute. Bethesda, MD.

27. Cold Spring Harbor Laboratory. "Phage Courses Begin at Cold Spring Harbor". Library & Archives. http://library.cshl.edu/resources/library-newsletter/161-2012-10-newsletter-2/331-phage-courses-begin-at-cold-spring-harbor . Accessed April 18, 2021.

28. Hollaender, A., Sansome E. R., Zimmer, E., Demerec, M., April 1945, "Quantitative Irradiation Experiments with Neurospora crassa. II. Ultraviolet Irradiation", American Journal of Botany 32(4):226–235; see http://www.estherlederberg.com/Papers.html

29. "Biological Effects of Radiation." Nuclear Regulatory Commission. Reactor Concept Manual https://www.nrc.gov/reading-rm/basic-ref/students/for-educators/09.pdf

30. HERSHEY, A D, and M CHASE. "Independent functions of viral protein and nucleic acid in growth of bacteriophage." The Journal of general physiology vol. 36,1 (1952): 39-56. doi:10.1085/jgp.36.1.39

31. "Pfizer-BioNTech COVID-19 Vaccine EUA Fact Sheet for Recipients and Caregivers." Centers for Disease Control. Access Date: 30, April, 2021.

https://www.cdc.gov/coronavirus/2019-ncov/vaccines/different-vaccines/Pfizer-BioNTech.html

32. National Center for Biotechnology Information. "PubChem Compound Summary for CID 24203, Disodium hydrogen phosphate" PubChem, https://pubchem.ncbi.nlm.nih.gov/compound/Disodium-hydrogen-phosphate. Accessed 1 May, 2021.

33. Carlson, Elof Axel (1981). Genes, radiation, and society: the life and work of H. J. Muller. Ithaca, N.Y: Cornell University Press. ISBN 978-0-8014-1304-9.

34. Beale, G. H. (1982). "Tracy Morton Sonneborn. 19 October 1905-26 January 1981". Biographical Memoirs of Fellows of the Royal Society. 28: 537–574. doi:10.1098/rsbm.1982.0021. JSTOR 769910

35. "James Dewy Watson." Indiana University. Access Date: 1, May, 2021. https://honorsandawards.iu.edu/awards/honoree/157.html

36. "James D. Watson." Cold Spring Harbor Laboratory. Access Date: 1, May, 2021. https://www.cshl.edu/giving/double-helix-medals-dinner/past-dhmd/2008-2/james-d-watson/

37. "James Watson: The most controversial statements made by the father of DNA." Independent. Access Date: 1, May, 2021. https://www.independent.co.uk/news/science/james-watson-racism-sexism-dna-race-intelligence-genetics-double-helix-a8725556.html

38. Statement by Cold Spring Harbor Laboratory addressing remarks by Dr. James D. Watson in "American Masters: Decoding Watson". Cold Spring Harbor Laboratory. Access Date: 1, May, 2021. https://www.cshl.edu/statement-by-cold-spring-harbor-laboratory-addressing-remarks-by-dr-james-d-watson-in-american-masters-decoding-watson/

39. Tijo and Levan: "The chromosome number in man". Hereditas, 42: 1, 1956.

40. A. Kornberg, "DNA Synthesis". San Francisco: Freeman, 1974.

41. Ingram V.M. Specific chemical difference between the globins of normal human and sickle-cell anemia hemoglobin. Nature, 178: 792-794. 1956 [PubMed]

42. Withrock, Isabelle C et al. "Genetic diseases conferring resistance to infectious diseases." Genes & diseases vol. 2,3 247-254. 25 Feb. 2015, doi:10.1016/j.gendis.2015.02.008

43. "What You Should Know About Sickle Cell Anemia Fact Sheet." The Centers for Disease Control, Bethesda, MD. Date Accessed: 2, May, 2021. https://www.cdc.gov/ncbddd/sicklecell/documents/SCD-factsheet_What-is-SCD.pdf

44. McGann, Patrick T et al. "Sickle cell anemia in sub-Saharan Africa: advancing the clinical paradigm through partnerships and research." Blood vol. 129,2 (2017): 155-161. doi:10.1182/blood-2016-09-702324

45. Risk for COVID-19 Infection, Hospitalization, and

Death By Race/Ethnicity. The Centers for Disease Control, Bethesda, MD. Date Accessed: 2, May, 2021. https://www.cdc.gov/coronavirus/2019-ncov/covid-data/investigations-discovery/hospitalization-death-by-race-ethnicity.html

46. Meselson, M, and F W Stahl. "THE REPLICATION OF DNA IN ESCHERICHIA COLI." Proceedings of the National Academy of Sciences of the United States of America vol. 44,7 (1958): 671-82. doi:10.1073/pnas.44.7.671

47. Chen, Yibao et al. "Specific Integration of Temperate Phage Decreases the Pathogenicity of Host Bacteria." Frontiers in cellular and infection microbiology vol. 10 14. 4 Feb. 2020, doi:10.3389/fcimb.2020.00014

48. Barák, Imrich, and Katarína Muchová. "The role of lipid domains in bacterial cell processes." International journal of molecular sciences vol. 14,2 4050-65. 18 Feb. 2013, doi:10.3390/ijms14024050

49. Braley R, Chaffin WL. Variations in mRNA transcript levels of cell wall-associated genes of Saccharomyces cerevisiae following spheroplasting. FEMS Microbiol Lett. 1999 Dec 1;181(1):177-85. doi: 10.1111/j.1574-6968.1999.tb08842.x. PMID: 10564805.

50. Barenkamp SJ, St Geme JW 3rd. Genes encoding high-molecular-weight adhesion proteins of nontypeable Haemophilus influenzae are part of gene clusters. Infect Immun. 1994 Aug;62(8):3320-8. doi: 10.1128/IAI.62.8.3320-3328.1994. PMID: 8039903; PMCID: PMC302962.

51. Williams, Bryan J et al. "Bacteriophage HP2 of Haemophilus influenzae." Journal of bacteriology vol. 184,24 (2002): 6893-905. doi:10.1128/jb.184.24.6893-6905.2002

52. Lejeune, J., Gautier, M., Turpin, R. Etude des chromosomes somatiques de neuf enfants mongoliens. C R Acad Sci, 248: 1721-1722. 1959.

53. Ford, C.E., Miller O.J., Polani P.E., de Almeida, J.C., Briggs, J.H. A sex-chromosome anomaly in a case of gonadal dysgenesis (Turner's syndrome). Lancet, 1: 711-713. 1959.

54. Jacobs, P.A., Strong, J.A.. A case of human intersexuality having a possible XXY sex-determining mechanism. Nature, 183: 302-3.1959.

55. Guthrie, R. Blood Screening for Phenylketonuria. JAMA, 178:863. 1961.

56. Luria, S.E. The Recognition of DNA in Bacteria. Scientific American, 222:88-92. 1970.

57. Meselson M., Yuan R. DNA restriction enzyme from E. coli. Nature, 217 (134):1110-4. 1968.

58. Smith, H.O., Wilcox K.W. A restriction enzyme from Hemophilus influenzae. I. Purification and general properties. J Mol Biol, 51: 379-91. 1970.

59. Jackson D.A., Symons R.H., Berg P. Biochemical method for inserting new genetic information into DNA of Simian Virus 40: circular SV40 DNA molecules containing lambda phage genes and the galactose operon of Escherichia coli. Proc Natl Acad

Sci, 69(10): 2904-9 1972.

60. Cohen S.N., Chang A.C., Boyer H.W., Helling R.B. Construction of biologically functional bacterial plasmids in vitro. Proc Natl Acad Sci, 70(11):3240-4. 1973.

61. Berg P., Baltimore D., Boyer H.W., Cohen S.N., Davis R.W., Hogness D.S., Nathans D., Roblin R., Watson J.D., Weissman S., Zinder N.D. Letter: Potential biohazards of recombinant DNA molecules. Science, 185(148):303. 1974.

62. Morrow J.F., Cohen S.N., Chang A.C., Boyer H.W., Goodman H.M., Helling R.B. Replication and transcription of eukaryotic DNA in Escherichia coli. Proc Natl Acad Sci, 71(5):1743-7. 1974.

63. Maxam, A.M., Gilbert, W. A new method for sequencing DNA. Proc Natl Acad Sci, 74 (2): 560-4. 1977.

64. Sanger, F. and Coulson, A.R. A rapid method for determining sequences in DNA by primed synthesis with DNA polymerase. J Molec Biol, 94: 441-448. 1975.

65. Sanger, F., Air, G.M., Barrell, B.G., Brown, N.L., Coulson, A.R., Fiddes, C.A., Hutchison, C.A., Slocombe, P.M., Smith, M. Nucleotide sequence of bacteriophage phi X174 DNA. Nature, 265(5596): 687-95. 1977.

66. Chow, L.T., Roberts, J.M., Lewis, J.B., Broker, T.R. A map of cytoplasmic RNA transcripts from lytic

adenovirus type 2, determined by electron microscopy of RNA:DNA hybrids. Cell, 11(4): 819-36. 1977.

67. Berk, A.J., Sharp, P.A. Sizing and mapping of early adenovirus mRNAs by gel electrophoresis of S1 endonuclease-digested hybrids. Cell, 12(3): 721-32. 1977.

68. Berget, S.M., Sharp, P.A. A spliced sequence at the 5'-terminus of adenovirus late mRNA. Brookhaven Symp Biol, 29:332-44, 1977.

69. Roberts and Sharp won the 1993 Nobel Prize in Physiology or Medicine "for their discoveries of split genes".

70. Costantini F., Lacy E. Introduction of a rabbit beta-globin gene into the mouse germ line. Nature, 294(5836):92-4. 1981.

71. N&V: Hogan, B., Williams, J. Integration of foreign genes into the mammalian germ line: genetic engineering enters a new era. Nature, 294(5836):9-10. 1981.

72. Gordon, J.W., Ruddle, F.H. Integration and stable germ line transmission of genes injected into mouse pronuclei. Science, 214(4526):1244-6. 1981.

73. Rubin, G.M., Spradling A.C. Genetic transformation of Drosophila with transposable element vectors. Science, 218(4570):348-53. 1982.

74. Ramsay M. Yeast artificial chromosome cloning. Mol Biotechnol. 1994 Apr;1(2):181-201. doi: 10.1007/BF02921558. PMID: 7859160.

75. Watson, J.D., Jordan, E. The Human Genome Program at the National Institutes of Health. Genomics, 5: 654-56. 1989.

76. Yun, Sang-Im et al. "Bacterial Artificial Chromosomes: A Functional Genomics Tool for the Study of Positive-strand RNA Viruses." Journal of visualized experiments: JoVE ,106 e53164. 29 Dec. 2015, doi:10.3791/53164

77. Adams, M.D., Kelley, J.M., Gocayne, J.D., Dubnick, M., Polymeropoulos, M.H., Xiao, H., Merril, C.R., et al. Complementary DNA sequencing: expressed sequence tags and human genome project. Science, 252:1651-6. 1991.

78. Murray, J.C., Buetow, K.H., Weber, J.L., Ludwigsen, S., Scherpbier-Heddema, T., Manion, F., Quillen, J., et al. A comprehensive human linkage map with centimorgan density. Cooperative Human Linkage Center (CHLC). Science, 265:2049-54. 1994.

79. Fleischmann, R.D., Adams, M.D., White, O., Clayton, R.A., Kirkness, E.F., Kerlavage, A.R., Bult, C.J., et al. Whole-genome random sequencing and assembly of Haemophilus influenzae Rd. Science, 269: 496-512 1995.

80. Fraser, C.M., Gocayne, J.D., White, O., Adams, M.D., Clayton, R.A., Fleischmann, R.D., Bult, C.J., et al. The minimal gene complement of Mycoplasma genitalium. Science, 270: 397-403, 1995.

81. Dietrich, W.F., Miller, J., Steen, R., Merchant, M.A., Damron-Boles, D., Husain, Z., Dredge, R., et al. A

comprehensive genetic map of the mouse genome. Nature, 380: 149-52. 1996.

82. Hillier, L.D., Lennon, G., Becker, M., Bonaldo, M.F., Chiapelli, B., Chissoe, S., Dietrich, N., et al. Generation and analysis of 280,000 human expressed sequence tags. Genome Res, 6: 807-28. 1996.

83. Schuler, G.D., Boguski, M.S., Stewart, E.A., Stein, L.D., Gyapay, G., Rice, K., White, R.E. A gene map of the human genome. Science, 274: 540-6. 1996.

84. Holtzman, N.A., Murphy, P.D., Watson, M.S., Barr, P.A. Predictive genetic testing: From basic research to clinical practice. Science, 278: 602-5. 1997.

85. Ito, T., Tashiro, K., Muta,S., Ozawa, R., Chiba, T., Nishizawa, M., Yamamoto, K., Kuhara, S., Sakaki, Y. Toward a protein-protein interaction map of the budding yeast: a comprehensive system to examine two-hybrid interactions in all possible combinations between the yeast proteins. Proc Natl Acad Sci USA, 97(3):1143-1147. 2000.

86. Elbashir, S.M., Harborth, J., Lendeckel, W., Yalcin, A., Weber, K., Tuschl, T. Duplexes of 21-nucleotide RNAs mediate RNA interference in cultured mammalian cells. Nature, 411: 494-498. 2001.

87. Mauro, M.J., Druker, B.J. STI571: targeting BCR-ABL as therapy for CML. Oncologist, 6: 233-238. 2001.

88. Waterson, R.H., Lindblad-Toh, K., Birney, E,. Rogers, J., et al. Initial sequencing and comparative analysis of the mouse genome. Nature, 420:520-562. 2002.

89. Organizing Evolution: Founding the Society for the Study of Evolution (1939-1950)

90. Author(s): Vassiliki Betty Smocovitis. Source: Journal of the History of Biology, Vol. 27, No. 2 (Summer, 1994), pp. 241-309 Published by: Springer Stable URL: http://www.jstor.org/stable/4331311

Chapter 5

1. Shampo, Marc A et al. “Sidney Altman--Nobel laureate for work with RNA.” Mayo Clinic proceedings vol. 87,10 (2012): e73. doi:10.1016/j.mayocp.2012.01.022

2. Doudna JA, Szostak JW. RNA-catalysed synthesis of complementary-strand RNA. Nature. 1989 Jun 15;339(6225):519-22. doi: 10.1038/339519a0. PMID: 2660003.

3. Ferre-d'Amare, A. R., Zhou, K. & Doudna, J. A. (1998) Nature 395 , 567–574. pmid:9783582

4. Kieft, J. S., Zhou, K., Jubin, R., Murray, M. G., Johnson, Y. N. L. & Doudna, J. A. (1999). J. Mol. Biol. 292 , 513–529. pmid:10497018

5. Wiedenheft, B., Sternberg, S. & Doudna, J. RNA-guided genetic silencing systems in bacteria and archaea. Nature 482, 331–338 (2012). https://doi.org/10.1038/nature10886

6. Jinek M, Chylinski K, Fonfara I, Hauer M, Doudna JA, Charpentier E. A programmable dual-RNA-guided

DNA endonuclease in adaptive bacterial immunity. Science. 2012 Aug 17;337(6096):816-21. doi: 10.1126/science.1225829. Epub 2012 Jun 28. PMID: 22745249; PMCID: PMC6286148.

7. "China's CRISPR babies: Read exclusive excerpts from the unseen research". Antonio Regalado. MIT Review. https://www.technologyreview.com/2019/12/03/131752/chinas-crispr-babies-read-exclusive-excerpts-he-jiankui-paper/

8. Doudna, Jennifer A.,, and Samuel H. Sternberg. A Crack in Creation: Gene Editing and the Unthinkable Power to Control Evolution. Boston: Houghton Mifflin Harcourt, 2017. Print.

9. Jones, Kate E.; Patel, Nikkita G.; Levy, Marc A.; Storeygard, Adam; Balk, Deborah; Gittleman, John L.; Daszak, Peter (February 21, 2008). "Global trends in emerging infectious diseases". Nature. 451 (7181): 990–993. Bibcode:2008Natur.451..990J. doi:10.1038/nature06536. ISSN 0028-0836. PMC 5960580. PMID 18288193.

10. Board on Life Sciences; Division on Earth and Life Studies; Committee on Science, Technology, and Law; Policy and Global Affairs; Board on Health Sciences Policy; National Research Council; Institute of Medicine. Potential Risks and Benefits of Gain-of-Function Research: Summary of a Workshop. Washington (DC): National Academies Press (US); 2015 Apr 13. 3, Gain-of-Function Research: Background and Alternatives. Available from:

https://www.ncbi.nlm.nih.gov/books/NBK285579/

11. Jessie Watters: The true origin of COVID (Transcript). Fox News. Published on May 8, 2021. https://video.foxnews.com/v/6253295880001#sp=show-clips

12. "The origin of COVID: Did people or nature open Pandora's box at Wuhan?" Nicholas Wade Published on May 5, 2021. The Bulletin of the Atomic Scientists. https://thebulletin.org/2021/05/the-origin-of-covid-did-people-or-nature-open-pandoras-box-at-wuhan/

13. Charles Calisher, Dennis Carroll, Rita Colwell, Ronald B Corley, Peter Daszak, Christian Drosten, Luis Enjuanes, Jeremy Farrar, Hume Field, Josie Golding, Alexander Gorbalenya, Bart Haagmans, James M Hughes, William B Karesh, Gerald T Keusch, Sai Kit Lam, Juan Lubroth, John S Mackenzie, Larry Madoff, Jonna Mazet, Peter Palese, Stanley Perlman, Leo Poon, Bernard Roizman, Linda Saif, Kanta Subbarao, Mike Turner. "Statement in support of the scientists, public health professionals, and medical professionals of China combatting COVID-19". The Lancet, Volume 395, Issue 10226, 2020, Pages e42-e43, ISSN 0140-6736, https://doi.org/10.1016/S0140-6736(20)30418-9. (https://www.sciencedirect.com/science/article/pii/S0140673620304189)

14. The Origins of SARS-CoV-2. The World Health Organization. https://www.who.int/health-topics/coronavirus/origins-of-the-virus

Chapter 6

1. Ute V. Solloch, Kathrin Lang, Vinzenz Lange, Irina Böhme, Alexander H. Schmidt, Jürgen Sauter. Frequencies of gene variant CCR5-Δ32 in 87 countries based on next-generation sequencing of 1.3 million individuals sampled from 3 national DKMS donor centers,

2. Human Immunology, Volume 78, Issues 11–12, 2017, Pages 710-717, ISSN 0198-8859,

3. https://doi.org/10.1016/j.humimm.2017.10.001.

: The Geographic Spread of the CCR5 Δ32 HIV-Resistance Allele. Novembre J, Galvani AP, Slatkin M (2005) The Geographic Spread of the CCR5 Δ32 HIV-Resistance Allele. PLOS Biology 3(11): e339. https://doi.org/10.1371/journal.pbio.0030339 "Editing of CCR5 receptor gene to protect against HIV infection". Juan Pablo Maianti and David R. Lui. Harvard University (Assignee). Patent No.: 10745677. U.S. Patent and Trademark Office. https://patents.justia.com/patent/10745677

5. 4. Lugade AA, Bogner PN, Murphy TF, Thanavala Y. The role of TLR2 and bacterial lipoprotein in enhancing airway inflammation and immunity. Front Immunol. 2011 Apr 27;2:10. doi: 10.3389/fimmu.2011.00010. PMID: 22566801; PMCID: PMC3342052.

6. Godlewska R, Wiśniewska K, Pietras Z, Jagusztyn-Krynicka EK. Peptidoglycan-associated lipoprotein

(Pal) of Gram-negative bacteria: function, structure, role in pathogenesis and potential application in immunoprophylaxis. FEMS Microbiol Lett. 2009 Sep;298(1):1-11. doi: 10.1111/j.1574-6968.2009.01659.x. Epub 2009 May 21. PMID: 19519769.

7. HrrF Is the Fur-Regulated Small RNA in Nontypeable Haemophilus influenzae

8. Santana EA, Harrison A, Zhang X, Baker BD, Kelly BJ, et al. (2014) HrrF Is the Fur-Regulated Small RNA in Nontypeable Haemophilus influenzae. PLOS ONE 9(8): e105644. https://doi.org/10.1371/journal.pone.0105644

9. Ratnayake G, Bain AL, Fletcher N, Howard CB, Khanna KK, Thurecht KJ. RNA interference to enhance radiation therapy: Targeting the DNA damage response. Cancer Lett. 2018 Dec 28;439:14-23. doi: 10.1016/j.canlet.2018.09.011. Epub 2018 Sep 18. PMID: 30240587. "'Sonic attacks' suffered by US diplomats likely caused by microwave energy, government study says". Jamie Crawford, CNN. https://www.cnn.com/2020/12/05/health/head-injuries-us-diplomats-government-study/index.html

10. "An Assessment of Illness in U.S. Government Employees and Their Families at Overseas Embassies". National Academies of Sciences. https://www.nap.edu/read/25889/chapter/1

Chapter 7

1. "Bill Gates, America's Largest Farm Owner". The Land Report. https://landreport.com/2021/01/bill-gates-americas-top-farmland-owner/

2. "The Wealthy flooded these four suburbs during the pandemic." Business Insider. March 19, 2021. https://www.businessinsider.com/wealthy-move-to-vacation-towns-long-term-during-pandemic-2021-2

3. "The wealthy invested in 'hidden gem' locations during the pandemic". Business Insider. May 5, 2021. https://www.businessinsider.com/luxury-real-estate-investing-salt-lake-city-dallas-migration-during-pandemic-2021

4. Bill & Melinda Gates Foundation Committed Grants to Cold Spring Harbor Laboratory https://www.gatesfoundation.org/about/committed-grants?q=cold%20spring%20harbor

5. Cold Spring Harbor Laboratory Receives $10 Million for Research Fund. Philanthropy News. June 9, 2015. https://philanthropynewsdigest.org/news/cold-spring-harbor-laboratory-receives-10-million-for-research-fund

6. Final Report DE-EE0005380 Assessment of Offshore Wind Farm Effects on Sea Surface,

7. Subsurface and Airborne Electronic Systems. Prepared by The University of Texas at Austin for The Department of Energy. September 30, 2003.

https://www.osti.gov/servlets/purl/1096175/

8. "Biden wants to move energy offshore, but choppy seas ahead". The Washington Post. May 8, 2021. https://www.washingtonpost.com/nation/2021/05/08/biden-wants-move-energy-offshore-choppy-seas-are-ahead/

9. "Ransomware attack leads to shutdown of major U.S. pipeline system". The Washington Post. May 8, 2021. https://www.washingtonpost.com/business/2021/05/08/cyber-attack-colonial-pipeline/

10. How Mark Zuckerberg spends his wealth. Business Insider. April 19, 2021. https://www.businessinsider.com/facebook-mark-zuckerberg-net-worth-priscilla-chan-2017-10

11. "Facebook removes faith-based website for 'misleading' coronavirus information. The Washington Post. May 7, 2021. https://www.washingtonpost.com/religion/facebook-ban-lifesite-covid/2021/05/07/638a4768-af48-11eb-acd3-24b44a57093a_story.html

Made in the USA
Monee, IL
04 November 2026

67381373R00118